D1244866

Foot Soldiers

Foot Soldiers

Stories from the Breast Cancer 3-Day Walk

Deborah Douglas, M.D.

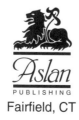

Aslan
PUBLISHING
Fairfield, CT

Aslan Publishing
2490 Black Rock Turnpike, #342
Fairfield, CT 06825
Please contact the publisher for a free catalog.
Phone: **203/372-0300**
Fax: **203/374-4766**
www.aslanpublishing.com

Library of Congress Cataloging-in-Publication Data

Douglas, Deborah, M.D.
  Foot soldiers : stories from the Breast Cancer 3-Day Walk / Deborah
Douglas.
      p. cm.
  Includes bibliographical references and index.
  ISBN 0-944031-24-2 (alk. paper)
  1. Breast—Cancer—Popular works. 2. Breast—Cancer—Patients—
United States—Biography. 3. Fund raising—United States. I. Title.

RC280.B8D667 2006
362.196'99449'00922—dc22
                                    2006010965

Editing by Joanne Shwed (www.backspaceink.com)
Book design by Dianne Schilling
Cover design by Miggs Burroughs
Printing by R.R. Donnelley
Printed in the USA

to the caregivers

Acknowledgements

I've heard that if a goose becomes injured, the other members of the flock will encircle and protect it until it is either able to fly again or until it perishes.

Were it not for many people—my mom and younger sisters; the people I worked with at Southeast Baptist Hospital; the members of Laurel Heights United Methodist Church; the teachers, staff, and other parents at St. Anthony Catholic School; three attorneys at my late husband's law firm; my husband's secretary, Tita Scott; and my friends, Michael Hardwick, Jean Holt, M.D., Jane Kline, Phil Kline, M.D., Scott and Barbara Lyford, Bernard Palmer, M.D., Scott and Priscilla Sowell, V. René Rone, M.D., and Al and Linda Ybarra (and many unnamed others, of course)—I could never have reached the threshold of this or, for that matter, any other project. Like an injured animal, I often shunned these people. Still, they remained within earshot, eager to help if I asked. My gratitude to this circle is incalculable. Words cannot begin ...

In Chapter 5, I tell how I came to be diagnosed with breast cancer. Dr. Beth Engelsgjerd, a gynecologist friend from medical school, was the first to insist on a biopsy of the palpable mass that had been dismissed by other doctors. Had I continued to listen to the others instead of my friend, Beth ...

In nearly every chapter, I mention Barbara Jo and Bob ("Dr. Bob") Kirshbaum. It's written elsewhere but it bears repeating: I could not have completed this project were it not for their help and encouragement and love. Yes, *love.* That is not too strong a word for what they showed me and for what I feel for them.

Dr. Sharon Wilks, medical oncologist and founder of the Alamo City Breast Cancer Council (www.acbcc.org), took time away from her busy clinical practice, her numerous volunteer patient advocacy activities, and her family to review the manuscript. Her suggestions not only clarified and updated the medical information, they steered me away from substantial embarrassment.

My women physicians' writing group—Drs. Beth Engelsgjerd, Christine Littlefield, Margaret Neiheisel, Deborah McNabb, V. René Rone, Cathy Spadaccini, and Sheila Swartzman—and our writing teacher, Marylyn Croman, waded through first drafts of some of the material and never, ever sneered when I stumbled. Their suggestions spared me still more embarrassment.

Joanne Shwed of Backspace Ink (www.backspaceink.com) provided top-shelf prepress and postproduction editing; Dianne Schilling designed a beautiful and elegant text; Miggs Burroughs designed a cover worthy of cradling the stories inside—no small task; Barbara and Harold Levine of Aslan Publishing (www.aslanpublishing.com) shaped all these pieces into a book on which I am honored to have my name.

I must mention my children: son, Andrew; daughter, Jessica; and son-in-law, David. My chief reason for writing or, for that matter, striving to accomplish anything meaningful, is because I love them so deeply. They are my beacons.

And then, of course, there is Tom. Sweet, gentle Thomas Fisher. We were broken and bruised when we found each other. In desperation, we grabbed the other's hand and held on for dear life, and, *my word*, how very dear that life has turned out to be. He became my safe harbor; he allowed me to become his. For that—for Tom—I am most grateful of all.

Foreword

An important way that cancer survivors address their dilemma is to tell their stories to others. Indeed, the utility of exchanging stories has been shown to benefit both the storyteller and their audience. In an important study, psychosocial researchers Yaskowich and Stam (1) used the narrative accounts of cancer patients' illnesses to derive a framework for exploring how cancer patients adjust and adapt. Through the stories of patients, the researchers found that a cancer diagnosis often comes with disrupted feelings of fit, which precipitates a renegotiation of personal identity and sense of purpose. Their qualitative data went on to show that the feelings of psychological "disconnect" resulting from bodily changes and other cancer-related events can be successfully mitigated through self-reflection and "biographical work." These efforts often bring forth a new and empowered sense of self. As for the audience, they note that "narratives become narrative only insofar as we find that they are our stories, too."

So it is with the stories in *Foot Soldiers: Stories from the Breast Cancer 3-Day Walk*. Author and breast cancer survivor, Deborah Douglas, M.D., gathered narratives while walking in all 10 of the 2004 Susan G. Komen/National Philanthropic Trust Breast Cancer 3-Day events. In each chapter of *Foot Soldiers*, we are introduced to new people and hear their stories. Time and again, we recognize our own fears, frustrations, concerns, and reactions in their voices. We also come to understand that the particular way in which a person deals with cancer is shaped by personal history, roles in family and work, stage in life, and the particulars of the medical diagnosis itself.

Advances in science, technology, and medicine have greatly improved cancer detection and treatment. The growing numbers of cancer survivors in the United States—now over 10 million—reflect this progress. Despite these advances, we are just now beginning to critically evaluate quality of life after cancer. The National Cancer Institute's Office of Cancer Survivorship and cancer centers like Memorial Sloan-Kettering, Dana-Farber, and M.D. Anderson, to name just a few, are actively pursuing clinical research to better understand the needs of new and long-term survivors. These needs are crisply articulated in the voices of the contributors to *Foot Soldiers*. Indeed, their narratives—narratives which emerged from brief, intense, and virtually random acquaintances with the author—provide valuable insight into the ways in which an individual's cancer experience is shaped by personal circumstances.

As a community psychologist, I appreciate the potential impact of events such as the Breast Cancer 3-Day as a vehicle for community building and for growing resources for cancer prevention and control; however, on another level, I also appreciate the opportunity that such events provide for individuals to share their stories. Since communities are complex, dynamic systems with their own environmental constraints and social characteristics, an individual's health and well-being can be either enhanced or compromised, depending on the quality of their community's resources and capacities. Indeed, as our population ages and chronic health problems such as cancer become more prevalent, community resources will be tested. Events such as the Breast Cancer 3-Day may become an increasingly valuable means for cancer survivors to create a supportive and trusting community—albeit temporary—in which to share their stories and to do the "biographical work" that is necessary for achieving an empowered sense of self.

David W. Lounsbury, Ph.D.
Department of Psychiatry & Behavioral Sciences
Memorial Sloan-Kettering Cancer Center
New York, New York

(1) Kyla M. Yaskowich and Henderikus J. Stam, "Cancer Narratives and the Cancer Support Group," *Journal of Health Psychology*, Vol. 8, No. 6, 720-737 (2003).

Table of Contents

Introduction

By all outward measures, our family was living happily ever after. My husband, Andy, and I had been married for 21 years. He was a defense attorney and I was a pathologist. We were rearing two outgoing, athletic children—a daughter, 15, and a son, 12—who were making all As and saying that they wanted to study law and medicine. Our nice house was in a nice Texas neighborhood, which was near the nice church that we regularly attended. The days of student loans, old Volkswagens, and grungy apartments were long past. Instead, our family was in a wide, grassy place, full of sunshine and possibilities. My metaphor, though, was about to be hit by a train.

Before daybreak on June 4, 1997, we were awakened by someone ringing the doorbell of our rented condominium on South Padre Island. We had arrived past my parents' bedtime the previous night, so I had not yet called to tell them our direct phone number. (Those were the days before ubiquitous cell phones.) The person at the door was a security guard. Among his duties was answering the front desk telephone between 11 PM and 6 AM. He asked if I was Dr. Douglas. When I nodded, he said, "You need to call your mother. Here's the phone number."

At that moment, my father was undergoing emergency surgery for what would turn out to be a highly malignant brain tumor. Although he survived the surgery, we were told that, even with aggressive treatment, he would probably be dead within a year. This was almost inconceivable because he had always been a trim, healthy physician. Besides, my father was supposed to live forever. Unfortunately, his diagnosis was only the first train wreck. The following February, Andy was diagnosed with metastatic rectal cancer. He was 46 years old. I remember beating my fists against a wall and screaming, "This can't be happening."

In August 1998, my father died after being bedridden for the last four months of his life. Almost exactly one year later, in August 1999, Andy died after being essentially bedridden for the last three months of his life. Less than two years later, yet another train appeared on the horizon: I was diagnosed with preinvasive breast cancer (ductal carcinoma *in situ* (DCIS). Since I was a pathologist (and supposedly a cancer expert), I was able to convince my beleaguered children that my outcome would be very different than their father and grandfather's. "My cancer is just a nuisance," I told them over and over.

Still, despite my excellent prognosis, my attitude toward cancer had already changed. In my professional role, I had once looked upon cancer as an intellectual challenge—something to be recognized, described, and labeled. Searching for and then studying cancer under the microscope had been the most interesting part of my job. Rare cancers and puzzling clinical manifestations of common cancers had been particularly fascinating, and I had shared these cases at the monthly Cancer Conferences of the hospital where I was chief-of-service. When I had come across one of these unusual cases, I had phoned my best friend (a pathologist who worked at a hospital across town) and bragged, "Guess what I've got?"

It was not that I was blind to the suffering caused by cancer prior to June 1997; it was just that I had never faced how cruel and unstoppable cancer could be. Cancer was no longer just a cover-glassed curiosity to be named and numbered in a pathology report. It had become a monster. In fact, by the time I was diagnosed, anxiety had erased any detachment I once had. After all, cancer had ripped holes in my family. Then, without a single risk factor in my history that would have warned me, it had attacked me, too. The threat to my children was the worst part. Their father and three of their grandparents had died of cancer, and I had been diagnosed at 48 years old. It was undeniable that cancer might strike them also.

Indirectly, it was anxiety that led me to write this book. In Chapter 6, I admit that the original intent of walking in all 10 of the 2004 Susan G. Komen/National Philanthropic Trust Breast Cancer 3-Day events was to prove that, in spite of my anxiety, I could still be adventurous—or, failing at that, I could at least quit wringing my hands long enough to walk 600 miles. It was only later that I decided to ask other survivors and co-survivors who were also participating to share their stories. I had anticipated that their stories would reflect the complexity of cancer diagnosis, treatment, and survivorship, but the surprise was the diversity of their coping tactics.

This diversity supported the important premise that individuals facing cancer will (and should be allowed to) rely on problem-solving strategies that have worked best for them in the past. Their stories also showed that participation in the 3-Day was not only a chance to "make a difference in the fight against breast cancer," but also a chance to battle negative emotions and struggle with personal conflicts that developed (or intensified) during their cancer experiences.

Before beginning, I need to make something clear: I didn't start out to teach anything important about battling cancer. Neither did the incredible people whom I walked beside. We simply told our stories. It turned out that, together, we teach a great deal.

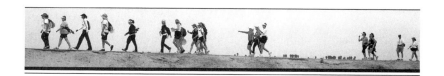

Chapter 1

Boston

July 30, July 31, and August 1, 2004

Because of the upcoming Democratic National Convention in Boston, the July 25, 2004, edition of *The New York Times* had a special 10-page insert called "Boston 2004." I skimmed some of the articles, including one about John Kerry's favorite pub, restaurant, and bicycle store, and skipped others, including a piece by Tom Hayden ("Advice From a Veteran of the Barricades"). Instead, I studied a color-coded map that showed Boston's points of interest in red and the assigned hotels of the state delegations in orange.

I noticed that delegates from Delaware and New York, for instance, were near Boston Common at the Park Plaza Hotel, and delegates from Michigan, New Mexico, Ohio, and West Virginia were staying at Democratic National Convention Headquarters at the Boston Sheraton. Massachusetts delegates had the Fairmount Copley Plaza Hotel all to themselves, and even South Dakota delegates—with their relatively meager three electoral votes—were within walking distance of FleetCenter from their orange block at the Wyndham Downtown. In contrast, Texas's assigned hotel was the Boston Logan Airport Hilton, which was so far away from FleetCenter that it only showed up on a circular inset map that overviewed traffic restrictions and road closings leading into the city.

My big, proud state's marginalization puzzled me until I read the front page of *The Boston Globe* on July 28, 2004. A story by staff writer Sarah Schweitzer, entitled "For Texas Delegates, a Lonely Role," began: "Texas is not a state accustomed to being treated small." Using Texas as "the most glaring example," she described the "status of states with little chance of a Democratic win in November" and showed how "the red states ... have been ignored in the goodies and attention lavished on 18 battleground states this week." This explained why the 232 delegates wearing Lone Star flag vests and flashing neon pins shaped like a cowboy boot had a view of the Boston Logan tarmac.

The local planners of the convention may have ignored the Texas delegation, but the local participants in the 3-Day seemed delighted that some of us had come all the way to Boston to support their cause. Three other Texans—two who lived in Nacogdoches (Loree McCary and DawnElla Rust) and one who had recently moved to Illinois (Jennie Collings)—were walking, too. Like strangers in a strange land, we recognized each other's drawls and twangs. Throughout the Boston 3-Day, we periodically huddled and compared funny stories. They, too, found that the locals were especially friendly toward the Texas delegation of the Boston 3-Day. We certainly were not "treated small."

It was not a native New Englander, however, but a transplanted Californian named Jennifer Stewart, 39, with whom I spent the most time at the Boston 3-Day. Jennifer had lived and worked in the Boston area for six years and loved New England. She could answer most of my questions about Boston but still maintained an outsider's eye for regional idiosyncrasies. While we walked the streets of Beverly, Salem, Willow Park, and, on the last day, Boston, she shared some of her observations about her adopted home and she shared her story.

Jennifer was 38 years old, rather than 40, which is the age for most women's first exam, when she had her first screening mammogram. This was because, unlike previous years when she had her annual appointment with a gynecologist, she checked the "yes" box for a family history of cancer. Six months before her appointment, her 88-year-old maternal grandmother had been diagnosed with breast cancer and had undergone a mastectomy. Jennifer's breast exam was normal that day—there were no masses, skin changes, or nipple discharge—but, "just to make us all rest easier," Jennifer's gynecologist ordered a mammogram.

A week later, Jennifer had a screening mammogram. The radiologist's scheduling clerk phoned the following day to ask Jennifer to return for a repeat mammogram. Jennifer was unconcerned because the technician had mentioned that a second mammogram was sometimes required, particularly in young women with dense breast tissue. After the second mammogram, the technician pointed out a questionable area within the shadowy image of her right breast. Still, Jennifer was not alarmed since she knew that the relative paucity of fat in young women's breasts sometimes complicated mammogram interpretation. Aware, also, that it was common for young women to undergo ultrasound imaging—particularly when a dense-appearing area needed to be distinguished from a fluid-filled cyst—Jennifer didn't worry when she was asked to return for an ultrasound. It never occurred to her that the questionable area might be cancer.

After the ultrasound examination, the radiologist reviewed the results of all the imaging studies with Jennifer. The dense area detected on the initial mammogram was confirmed by the second mammogram, and the ultrasound examination showed that the dense area was not a cyst but rather a mass. Although the radiologist reassured Jennifer that the mass was probably nothing to worry about, she referred (a still unalarmed) Jennifer to a surgeon. After examining Jennifer and reviewing the imaging studies, the surgeon recommended a needle-directed excisional biopsy. Again, Jennifer dismissed the notion that she might have cancer, reasoning that age was "on my side."

A week later, Jennifer underwent a needle localization of the breast mass, followed by an excisional biopsy under general anesthesia. A thin, sleeved wire (the "needle") was inserted into the breast mass, using the images on the ultrasound screen as a guide. When the sleeve was removed, a little bend at the end of the wire popped out, effectively anchoring the wire. A loose bandage was placed over the protruding end of the wire. This part of the procedure was done in the Radiology department by the radiologist, who was assisted by a radiology technician. Although the ultrasound exam itself was virtually painless (unlike a mammogram, sustained compression of the breast tissue is unnecessary for an ultrasound), Jennifer wryly described the needle localization as "loads of fun."

A short while later, when Jennifer was in the Operating Room under general anesthesia, the surgeon used the anchored wire as a guide for locating and excising (removing) the mass with a rim of uninvolved (normal-appearing) breast tissue. The tissue (with its anchored wire still in place) was put in a labeled container and sent to the Pathology department for routine examination.

"Routine examination" (as opposed to "frozen section examination," which will be described in the next chapter) means that biopsy tissue is processed in a machine prior to being examined under the microscope. Before being processed, the tissue undergoes a "gross examination," which means that the pathologist describes certain features of the tissue, such as its weight and size and the appearance of the cut surface after it has been sliced with a scalpel. If a discrete mass is visible, as it was in Jennifer's case, it is described and examined in detail. The pathologist's gross description of her biopsy tissue would have also mentioned the localizing wire in the report.

Before it is processed in the machine, the tissue to be examined under the microscope is cut into pieces (about 0.3 cm thick) and placed in labeled, perforated plastic boxes. These boxes are put in a metal basket that rotates through solutions in an automated tissue-processing machine, which is an overnight operation in most laboratories. After this step is finished, a histotechnologist prepares glass slides of the biopsy tissue and gives them to a pathologist for microscopic examination and preliminary reporting. In pathology-speak, these slides are the "routine stains."

If the pathologist sees a malignant lesion—either invasive cancer or ductal carcinoma *in situ* (DCIS)—sections of the tumor tissue undergo additional special studies, which help predict how aggressively the tumor will behave and whether or not the patient will benefit from hormonal treatment. These additional studies take at least several days and sometimes even a week or two. In Jennifer's case, it took several weeks for one assay to be repeated and confirmed by a central testing facility (Boston's Dana-Farber Cancer Institute). The results of this assay were critical since they determined whether Jennifer would benefit from chemotherapy. But I'm getting ahead of the story.

Jennifer was taken to the Recovery Room after the procedure, and the surgeon told the friend, who was waiting to drive Jennifer home from the hospital, that he didn't think it was cancer but the tissue was being examined by Pathology. The surgeon had other cases so the friend told Jennifer the good news after she recovered from anesthesia. It was not until she called the surgeon's office to confirm the date and time of the post-op visit that she became a little concerned. "I was pretty much under the assumption that I was just going in [to the surgeon's office] to have the steri-strips removed. I called on Tuesday and the nurse sounded a little strange. Something about her tone struck me as odd. I began to worry a little bit, but I told myself that I was just imagining it."

As a child, Jennifer became astute at recognizing the subtle cues that signaled impending mood swings in people, which evolved into a hyperacuity for sensing what she called people's "negativity." This ability proved particularly useful in her previous job position that involved personnel scheduling for an accounting firm. One of her assignments was to determine if an employee—one whom she may never have seen—was being forthright about, for instance, a request for additional time or manpower to complete a project. It was Jennifer's responsibility to determine the legitimacy of the request.

"Sometimes it involved me saying, not in so many words, 'I know what you're up to, and you're not going to pull this on me.' No matter how much good personal chemistry there is with the people you are scheduling, there is the potential for animosity. I ended up being the bad guy when they realized they had to work late to meet a deadline. I had a few of the managers get rather vocal when I reminded them that they were the ones who had told me that they could meet the deadline without extra help.One guy from Chicago actually yelled, 'F___ you,' and hung up on me. I nicknamed him Mr. Impulse Control Problem."

A few months after this interrupted phone call, she attended a meeting at her firm's Chicago office and met Mr. I.C. Problem. He wasn't at all what she had expected. He was a large, outgoing man, and she liked him very much. They became friends, and when she was later diagnosed with breast cancer, he was the one who informed the 10 or 12 people who needed to know the situation. Jennifer said, "He was very kind to me throughout the whole time, but not in a way that made me think he felt sorry for me. He'd call me up and say, 'What's up, Stewie?' That's the nickname some people use at work for me. And, when I was one of the 30 people in my department who got laid off, he told me he thought it stunk. I took an administrative assistant position with my company for a little less pay and a lot less stress, so I don't travel anymore, but he said that if I ever came to Chicago again, we could go to a baseball game. He's a sweet guy."

Jennifer's ability to read people was a valuable skill in career situations; however, she admitted that it might have caused her to prematurely veto potential relationships. Still, she couldn't ignore her intuitions. "Sometimes, I wish I hadn't gotten good at it [reading people]. When I pick up something I can't explain, other people don't always believe me. Once, when I expressed concern about a friend's fiancé, I was accused of being jealous. Everyone else thought he was hunky and charismatic, but I had such negative feelings about the guy that I had trouble being in the same room with him. It turned out that he was beating her." Jennifer almost imperceptibly shuddered when she said this.

The day following the disquieting phone conversation with the nurse, Jennifer went to the surgeon's office alone. When she was in the exam room, she undressed from the waist up and put on a johnny (a hospital gown). The nurse with whom Jennifer had spoken on the phone was in the exam room when the surgeon removed the steri-strips and examined the incision site. After he helped Jennifer sit up, he took her hands in his and said, "Jennifer, I don't want to beat around the bush. It turned out to be cancer. After you get dressed, we'll talk." He continued to hold her hands while she absorbed the information and, only then, left the exam room so that she could get dressed.

Jennifer was so stunned that she remembered very little about the conversation that followed other than that the tumor was invasive, but small (0.7 cm), and that the surgical margins were clear of tumor involvement. She also remembered hearing that she would need a lymph node biopsy and that she was being referred to a medical oncologist (a cancer specialist). Before she left his office, the surgeon said he understood that she might be having difficulty retaining all the information, particularly since the cancer diagnosis was so unanticipated, and encouraged her to call back if she had questions or needed clarification.

Jennifer didn't start crying until she got on the bus to go back to her apartment. Once home, she steadied herself before making two phone calls: the first to her parents in Virginia; the second to her supervisor to say that she would be a little late to work that morning. Less than two hours after learning that she had invasive breast cancer (and after pausing to have what she called "a good cry"), Jennifer Stewart took a shower, walked to the commuter rail station (the "T" platform), and went to work. When she arrived, she spoke with her boss and two of her closest co-workers, and then to the Human Resources department personnel to tell them that she had invasive breast cancer, but that she didn't yet know what treatment she would be receiving. After working the remainder of the day, she rode the "T" home, cooked dinner for herself, and logged onto her blog—"Cup and Saucer" (www.cupandsaucer.com)—to check comments about that morning's post.

Jennifer's blog (a personal Web site that is essentially an online journal) was already well visited when she was diagnosed with breast cancer in June 2003. In fact, in October 2003, while she was undergoing chemotherapy (and "bald as a billiard"), her blog had its 30,000th visitor since its inception 14 months earlier. In one of her posts, Jennifer described her blog's contents as "regularly scheduled general looniness and Bostonian hooha. Of which there is a vast and goofy supply." (Note: Jennifer's final "Cup and Saucer" entry was March 2005, but in January 2006, she returned to blogging with a new domain: www.jenstewart.com, which has the heading, "Jenny Sais Quoi: In search of less clutter, more quiet, and a really good cup of tea.")

On the opening page of "Cup and Saucer," she described herself this way: "Depending on who you ask, I'm either Jennifer, Jen, Jane or DeeDee ... I'm in my thirties, I'm klutzy, a Republican, a Catholic, a former English major, and a dedicated bookworm." Explaining why she established a blog, she wrote, "Why not? Okay, that's not the best of all possible answers, I guess. How about this: Because my friends and family are spread out all over the country (in some cases, all over the world), and this is an easy way for me to keep everyone abreast of what's up with me. That, and I like the blog venue for tossing my thoughts out there. And why 'cup and saucer,' you ask? Well, because I collect them, I love pretty much anything that can be served in 'em, and I just like the sound of the words. It's as simple or as complicated as that."

(Jennifer's choice for a blog name may have had something to do with a childhood incident that she described while we were walking together. When she was reading Frances Hodgson Burnett's *The Secret Garden,* she was confused by the phrase "go to tea." Her mother, in a good mood that day, prepared an English-style high tea, complete with cucumber sandwiches and toast with jelly.)

In her near-daily entries, she discussed everything from the pleasures of dining alone at her favorite restaurant (Lala Rokh) to the absurdity of a poster on the "T" platform that reads "Kahlua ... unleash it." She even posted the occasional open letter to someone with whom she had had contact. An excerpt from one of her posts, entitled "Cranky, Cranky, Cranky," read:

Dear Male Commuter,
At no time, and under no circumstances, should you place your crotch on my knee. There are some parts of strangers' anatomies with which I do not have any desire to become more closely acquainted, a couple of layers of clothing betwixt notwith-

standing. When faced with the dilemma of knocking your 567 lb. backpack into the commuter behind you or mounting my knee like an unrestained poodle, please choose a third option: remove your backpack, place it between your feet, stand up straight, and keep your privates off my patella.

For six weeks, Jennifer did not mention her diagnosis and treatment for breast cancer in her blog. In fact, not until after her surgery for removal of axillary (underarm) lymph nodes did she say anything and, only then, because "scrubbing the [cancer] details" from the posts while trying to "maintain context" was becoming problematical. In the entry entitled, "For the Sake of Context …," she wrote:

So, I think I'd just like to get it out in the open now, and then move on. That way, if I have a funny tale to tell about what the wacky lady in the radiology waiting room said about her dog, or how my oncologist reminds me of the farmer in "American Gothic" (truly he does … to a spooky degree), I won't have to sanitize the details of where I was and why. That said, my blog hasn't been a morose "here are my problems" blog up until now; it's been my "Gee, don't I have a goofy life?" blog with the occasional essay on things I ponder or enjoy (or both), and that's what I want it to continue being. But I know that, until I'm free and clear of the threat of cancer, things like radiation, scans, doctors, and (possibly, but hopefully not) chemo will be part of my daily life for months, and they will creep into various posts, here and there.

The first time Jennifer blogged about cancer, she still did not know the pathology results for the axillary lymph nodes that had been removed two days before. She also did not have the final results of a critical assay that was pending on the original biopsy tissue. In other words, she was awaiting information that would determine whether or not she needed chemotherapy. She ended her blog by listing three things that she had already learned from being sick. "Prayer is tremendously helpful—so if you're inclined, please feel free to pray for me …" Next, she wrote:

I'm really independent and no-frills, so lots of fussing and there-there-there-ing and hand-wringing make me nervous. So, um, don't do it, okay? Seriously. No fussing, no omigoshyoupoorthingyou-ing. I'm not a poor thing. My prognosis is exceedingly good, I'm in capable hands, and I'm otherwise pretty healthy. So no "poor Jen" stuff. Spend that currency on someone who really is in a world of hurt, and we'll both feel better (and so, probably, will the person who does actually need that level of there-there-ing).

Lastly, she urged her online readers to give her "a good swift kick in the pants" if they detected any self-pity, but that "the occasional pep talk" or "(clean!) joke" would be welcome. She ended the entry by promising to keep everyone informed about her progress "without dwelling unnecessarily on the whole ordeal."

As it turned out, the "ordeal" was somewhat more complicated and lengthy than Jennifer had initially anticipated. She soon learned that, although her axillary lymph nodes were negative for metastatic carcinoma, the cell membranes of her tumor had overexpression (excess amounts) of the glycoprotein *HER-2/neu* (often abbreviated as "*HER-2*"). This was a setback.

Since first described in 1984, the oncogene *HER-2/neu* (also called *c-erbB-2*) has been investigated in numerous clinical studies. In general, its overexpression has been linked with reduced survival in cancer patients; however, as Jennifer soon discovered, most of the completed clinical studies with published results had evaluated patients with relatively advanced cancer (Stages III and IV). (Note: Studies which have since matured that include patients with Stage I and Stage II disease indicate that overexpression of *HER-2* carries a worse prognosis, regardless of stage at diagnosis.)

She said, "I went searching on the Internet to see what I could find out about it, and it was so disheartening. There was not any information about Stage I or Stage II disease. It was all about Stage III and Stage IV, and the prognosis was very bad, and I was like, o-h-h-h-h-h, n-o-o-o. But, fortunately, I talked to a medical oncologist in Boston with whom I had a mutual friend. He explained it to me in a way that didn't freak me out. He put my mind at rest."

Despite the fact that Jennifer's primary tumor was small and her axillary lymph nodes were negative, both her local medical oncologist—the one who reminded her of "American Gothic"—and the oncologist at Dana-Farber Cancer Institute, from whom she sought a second opinion, recommended adjuvant chemotherapy because of her tumor's overexpression of *HER-2*. ("Adjuvant" is the general term for the chemotherapy treatment that is given after surgical removal of all detectable disease. Its intent is to ferret out and kill any stray tumor cells that might linger, waiting for an opportunity to multiply and develop into a local or regional recurrence or a distant metastasis.)

To facilitate administration of the intravenous chemotherapy, her doctors also recommended that she have placement of a portacath (or mediport catheter). This is a small, biscuit-shaped device with a puncturable membrane (a port) on one surface and a slender tube (a catheter) extending from the edge. The device is inserted just under the skin in an envelope created in the soft tissue of the chest, about 3 to 4 cm from the bottom edge of the collarbone. The catheter is threaded into the subclavian vein and through the superior vena cava to its junction with the right atrium of the heart. When chemotherapy treatment is finished, the portacath is removed. Despite sounding rather grisly, both the placement and removal are relatively simple surgical procedures and are usually done as outpatient procedures rather than in the Operating Room of a hospital.

When a patient needs chemotherapy treatment or needs to have blood drawn for laboratory tests, the needle is inserted through the chest skin and into the membrane of the portacath rather than into the arm, like most intravenous procedures. It is not only less painful for the patient when a portacath is used, but it also spares the patient's veins from the cumulative effects of multiple needle sticks and repeated exposures to caustic chemotherapy agents (drugs). In addition, some types of chemotherapy cause severe damage (functionally, a third-degree burn) of the skin and soft tissue if there is leakage from a peripheral (arm or hand) vein. A portacath virtually precludes this serious complication.

Over the objections of well-meaning friends who insisted on the superiority of Dana-Farber, Jennifer decided to receive her treatment at nearby Melrose-Wakefield Hospital. The medical oncologist at Dana-Farber, who offered a second opinion, was very knowledgeable but variably called her either "Janet" or "Jessica." Overall, she felt "like a number" at that institution. In contrast, her doctors, the nurses, and the staff at Melrose-Wakefield knew her name. And, since she didn't own a car, traveling to Dana-Farber would have also been difficult.

Jennifer was scheduled to receive four cycles of doxorubicin hydrochloride (Adriamycin®) and cyclophosphamide (Cytoxan®) as adjuvant combination chemotherapy. From the outset, she knew that she would lose her hair, but this prospect didn't particularly bother her. What did sadden her was the likelihood of chemotherapy causing premature menopause. She had hoped that she might marry and bear a child before her natural menopause. "Until that point, a window of opportunity still existed for me to have children. Honestly, that [loss of fertility] bothered me more than anything else."

Still, Jennifer blogged on, without a whiff of self-pity in any of her posts. In fact, in the middle of chemotherapy, she wrote the following entry entitled, "Whatcha See Is, Well, Whatcha Get":

> *I know this should be a no-brainer, but when someone asks me how I'm doing, and I reply "Fine!" or "Peachy!" or "Great!" it really is okay to believe me, you know. Because I'm telling the truth. What you see is what you get. If I'm having an angst-ridden day, trust me: you'll know. I'm crabby, tired, distraught, it won't be a mystery. Likewise, if I'm smiling, upbeat, full of energy, well, that's the real deal, too. I'm really just not grasping these folks who ask, "How are you doing?" and, when I reply "Fine, thanks!" feel the need to inform me that I'm lying. Or need to let me know, in conspiratorial tones, that they know I'm not really fine, but that I'm really "just trying to be brave." People. Please. You credit me with more complexity than I possess, to say nothing of assuming that I have such respect for your delicate sensibilities that I'd martyr myself emotionally rather than let you believe there are unhappy people in the world and that I might be one of them. Meanwhile, I'm having a pretty darned good day, so if you don't mind, I'd like to go back to enjoying that, without being encumbered with all these haphazard (and not terribly accurate) attempts at omniscience.*

Jennifer continued to refuse to feel sorry for herself even after she developed a frightening complication during chemotherapy. Her portacath worked well for the first cycle of chemotherapy; however, three weeks later, when it was time for the second cycle, the portacath malfunctioned. She was immediately sent to the Radiology department for an imaging study (a "port study") to determine if a blood clot was blocking the catheter tubing. As she waited alone in the hospital hallway to undergo the procedure, she became truly frightened for the first time. Despite her anxiety, Jennifer still had a sense of humor: "I sat there thinking, I know breast cancer doesn't grow very fast, but this blood clot—it could just cut loose and *go*. What if I were sleeping? Is my house clean? Oh, God, I can't die with a dirty house."

Her surgeon happened to be in the hospital while she was waiting for the procedure. When he learned that she was there for a port study, he came to the Radiology department and, until she was wheeled in for the study, sat in a chair beside her and held her hand. Jennifer said that this simple gesture was enormously comforting. Unfortunately, the port study confirmed that a blood clot had developed in the vein, making the portacath unusable. Later that day, when the surgeon learned the results of the study, he called her at home. He knew how frightened Jennifer was, so he told her, "If I thought you needed to stay in the hospital for observation, you'd be here for observation. The clot will dissolve all by itself. You will be okay." Even though she was relieved to hear this, Jennifer blogged several months later that, in retrospect, this complication was the low point of her ordeal:

> ... I finally had a meltdown. I was not used to my body betraying me—in fact, I was unused to my body doing anything but being sturdy and healthy. And, so, I cried quite a bit and struggled with being afraid. I thank God enormously for the friends and family who comforted and buoyed me during this time, because I know I could not have handled it alone.

Among the friends to whom she was referring were members of Sacred Hearts in Malden, where she worshiped. She has not always been a Catholic. In fact, it was after she moved to Boston, when she was in her early 30s, that she attended parish classes and was formally confirmed. Becoming a Catholic was part of an emotionally complicated departure from the evangelical church in which she was reared and, in a very real sense, a part of establishing ideological independence from her parents—a process that had started years before.

When Jennifer was 20 years old and majoring in English at Riverside Community College, she worked for a group of psychologists. One of the requirements of the employees was to undergo psychological evaluation and a few counseling sessions. For the first time, Jennifer— who, by the way, is one of the most psychologically intact women I have ever met—acknowledged (and subsequently expressed) anger about her family's dynamics. She came to believe that many of her family's internal struggles were certainly aggravated, if not caused by, their church's rigid fundamentalism.

Although Jennifer did not reject her parents, she withdrew from the organized focus of their religiosity, leaving behind a childhood and young adulthood that had been riveted to the church. She did not attend worship services for a decade. However, when she moved to Boston, she began worshiping again, attending first Episcopalian and then Catholic services. Religion became an important part of her life, albeit with a different compass setting than before.

One of her former bosses served as her confirmation sponsor. Knowing about Jennifer's cooking skills and domestic bent, he joked that instead of St. Catherine of Sienna, she should choose St. Martha (as in Martha Stewart) for her confirmation name. Because of his history of concocting elaborate practical jokes, she was concerned that he might actually blurt out "Martha" during the service, just to get her tickled.

Conversations with Jennifer often drifted toward food. So did her blog entries, which, in addition to describing food, also mentioned other sensual things, like chilly autumn weather, her yellow chenille bathrobe, and the rapturous solitude between 4:30 and 5:30 in the morning—her preferred time for blogging and sipping a cup of tea. These other little pleasures notwithstanding, she readily volunteered, "I'm all about food."

One of my favorite memories of the Boston 3-Day indirectly resulted from her food antennae. On our way into camp on Day 2, she spotted a Dairy Queen in the distance. Jennifer is a big fan of DQ, as am I, so even after walking all day, taking showers, eating dinner, and cheering in the last of the walkers arriving in camp, we walked another half-mile to Dairy Queen. Over a root beer float (hers) and a butterscotch sundae (mine), we laughed and talked about everything from her Ozark aunts' unusual names (Xlee, Fern, and Bernice, pronounced like "furnace") to tamoxifen's side effects. We were so absorbed in conversation that we missed a turn and ended up walking several extra blocks.

After she finished college and worked for a few years, Jennifer considered going to culinary school; however, by then, she had become friends with two chefs through her waitressing and catering department jobs. She changed her mind about culinary school after she saw the effects of day-long food preparation on the chefs' attitudes about eating. "When they got home, they were so sick of cooking that they ate Cap'n Crunch® out of a box. Hanging over the sink. By the fist. That looked miserable to me."

In contrast, she talked about how much she enjoys shopping for ingredients and cooking. She also enjoys reading and writing about food. (She once wrote restaurant reviews for an online magazine.) She especially enjoys cooking for small gatherings, and comforts herself with fresh, healthy, well-prepared food and the ever-present cup of tea. When she was taking anticoagulants (blood thinners) for her portacath (and, after that clotted, her PICC line—a peripherally inserted central catheter), there were dietary restrictions of foods rich in vitamin K because of its interference with the action of blood thinners. These restrictions included some of her favorite foods like broccoli and dark, leafy green vegetables. She attributed some of her temporary weight gain during chemotherapy treatment to her inability to eat her favorite low-calorie foods.

Jennifer gained 20 pounds during treatment, which was very distressing to her. First of all, the weight gain was associated with an increase in her serum cholesterol to a level that, had it persisted, would have required that she take a lipid-lowering agent.

Her ability to lose the extra pounds after finishing chemotherapy was partly because she could resume her usual eating habits, but it was also due to the training necessary to participate in the Boston 3-Day. In December 2003, on the day of her last chemotherapy treatment, she asked her oncologist if it would be safe for her to begin training for the walk. She had vowed that, if he said it was okay, she would raise the necessary funds and participate. When he gave her medical clearance, she was off and walking. And fund raising.

Over the next eight months, she raised nearly $7,500 from 141 donors. (On Day 3, she wore a t-shirt with her contributors' names on it.) Despite the sometimes staggering fatigue associated with the seven weeks of radiation treatment that followed combination chemotherapy, and the hot flashes associated with tamoxifen treatment, she continued to train. In the opening page to the "Cup and Saucer" breast cancer page, Jennifer blogged: "Joining the 3-Day walk is, for me, about two things: One, it is about raising funds to further research, education, screening, and treatment for others facing this disease. But it's also about reclaiming my body and getting back on the healthy track ... I view this event as a means to becoming 'normal.'"

Her training walks started out at less than a mile, but she gradually increased the distance. By spring 2004, her weekend walks lasted several hours. It was during one of her long walks that she met some members of Team Wild Women Outfitters (now called Team Wild Women Originals or "Team WWO"), who were also training for the 3-Day. They soon recruited Jennifer.

_____

The co-captains of Team WWO are Karen Rudnick of Lexington and Lyn Ostberg of West Roxbury. These two women met in 2002 while preparing for their first Boston 3-Day walk. The following year, they volunteered as training leaders to help others prepare for long-distance walks and, with the support of Lisa and Terry Austin, co-owners of the retail store, Wild Women Outfitters, in Arlington, Massachusetts, formed Team Wild Women Outfitters. (After the store closed, the team's name was modified.) The team steadily grew and, in 2004 alone, 183 members participated in long-distance walks—the Susan G. Komen 3-Day event and the Avon 2-Day event—and raised over half a million dollars. Their team's accomplishments were so remarkable that Thomas M. Menino, mayor of the City of Boston, proclaimed July 30, 2004 (the first day of the Boston 3-Day event) as "Wildly Walking for a Cure Day in the City of Boston."

The individual team members were easy to spot during the Boston 3-Day because of their flamingo-themed hats, extravagant costume jewelry, bright t-shirts, and pink feather boas. And, when two or more of them got together, something happened—not always wild, but always noisy and cheerful. They were often funny, too, although, perhaps, not always intentionally. One of the most memorable lines came from a Wild Woman as she stepped out of the porta-potty. With a troubled look, she announced to all of us who were waiting in line: "I have a wedgie that I can't find."

The Wild Women could also be inspiring, particularly if your feet were aching, you were exhausted, and it was near the end of the route on the third day of the event. Their excerpted marching words were:

3-Day walkers are the best. We raise money for the breast.
Make that cancer go away, so we can live another day.
Rise before the sun comes up to tell the world we won't give up.
3-Day walkers can't be beat. We have blisters on our feet.
3-Day walkers do appear to have muscles on their rear.
3-Day walkers are the best, fighting cancer of the breast.
Of this one thing we are sure, we'll keep walking 'til there's a cure.
I trained and trained for miles and miles with a group of women that are wild.
I couldn't have walked these 60 miles. I couldn't have done it without their smiles.

The members of Team WWO were largely responsible for setting the garrulous and team-spirited tone of the 2004 Boston 3-Day walk. They had help from the members of another Boston-area group, Men With Heart. Founded in 2002 by Paul Boulanger, Jack Burlingame, Scott Walters, and Matt Cushing, it has become the largest men-only team of its type. By 2004, they had raised well over $215,000 in the fight against breast cancer. Actually, the total raised was considerably more than that, since members of Men With Heart willingly shared their donation money at registration with other Boston-area teams and individuals who had not been able to raise the minimum $2,000 per walker required to enter a Breast Cancer 3-Day event. At other times, they wrote personal checks to cover the shortfalls.

Another way Men With Heart members supported the event was by lugging backpacks filled with supplies that other walkers might need along the route. Laminated inventories were on the outside of the backpacks, listing things like blister packs, clean socks, candy, Motrin®, cough drops, duct tape, sunscreen, and lip balm. A yellow circle in the left-hand corner of the inventory sheet declared: "New for 2004! Tampons." (Only men who are secure in their manhood would do that.)

Men With Heart members also functioned as cheerleaders for the women walkers. Along the route, they chatted, serenaded, made us laugh, and, of course, doled out supplies. On Days 1 and 2, they formed receiving lines at the end of the route, singing "Pretty Woman" and applauding as tired women straggled in. I think I speak for most of the women when I say that those men were appreciated beyond measure for being willing to walk 60 miles with us in order to support our cause. And to do it with panache.

I was lucky that my tent site assignment was near two members of Men With Heart. My assigned tent mate, Barbara Jo Kirshbaum, was staying at a nearby hotel with her husband, Bob, so I had the tent to myself. That night, as I was shifting around, trying for the first time since college to get comfortable in a tent—or, for that matter, on anything besides a good mattress with clean sheets—I overheard this conversation between two Men With Heart members:

"Are you naked in there?"

"No, I'm not naked."

"Well, believe me, if you're naked in there, I'm not sleeping with you."

"Whassa matter? Male love is a beautiful thing."

"Hey, everyone! Jimmy's naked!"

"I'm *not* naked. I'm just trying to find out a good way to get comfortable here."

"I'm going to make a wall between us, so we won't wake up … you know."

"You're not naked, are you?"

"No! I'm not naked."

(mumble, mumble)

"It's going to be really fun spending the night with you, laughing and giggling."

"Did you take a shower?"

"Was I supposed to?"

"Maybe I'll sleep outside the tent."

"There are mosquitoes out the wazoo, and it may rain."

"It's not going to rain."

"Yeah, but it's gonna get all dewy."

(mumble, mumble)

"Where's my … Someone stole my panties!"

"Nobody wants your panties."

"How would you know if someone wants my panties?"

(mumble, mumble)

"I have a cold. Will you sniff these shorts and see if they're clean?"

"I don't have to sniff them. I can tell from here."

(mumble, mumble)

"What side's your vent on?"

"I dunno. Why do you wanna know?"

"Well, you're gonna want to sleep with your head down that way."

"I was supposed to brush my teeth, too? Jeez. I'm not sleeping with a naked guy who's wanting me to shower *and* brush my teeth."

"I'm not naked."

"So what are you wearing?"

"Pink panties."

"Lemme see."

"Uh, uh."

(mumble, mumble)

"Get your hand off my side."

"That's not my hand, big boy."

Soon all the women within earshot were laughing, which was, of course, the point. Finally, around 9 PM—the more or less official time to quiet down, turn off cell phones, and go to sleep—one of the men offered to sing us a lullaby. It must have worked because that's the last thing I remember.

It wasn't long, though, before I awoke for the first of what turned out to be three times that night, slipped on my flip-flops, put on my cap with the reading light clipped to the visor, heaved myself to a half-standing position, painfully stepped out of my tent, and shuffled to the porta-potty. (The reading light was a gift from one of my little sisters, which turned out to be a brilliant alternative to a hand-held flashlight when visiting a dark porta-potty in the middle of the night.) Had my urinary bladder not forced me to get up and hobble around several times during the night, I might have been too stiff and sore to dress and go to breakfast at 5 AM on Saturday morning. At 6:30 AM, when the course opened, I was feeling—if not ready for line dancing—ready to walk at my customary 2.5-mile-per-hour pace.

There was another reason that I was also relieved, so to speak, to be getting up in the middle of the night. According to the 3-Day safety video, which all participants were required to watch, getting up at least once in the middle of the night to pee indicated that I was drinking enough fluids. The video described how to recognize and avoid dehydration and hyponatremia, stressed the importance of pacing yourself and pausing once an hour to stretch, and showed how to signal a passing "sweep" van or other 3-Day vehicle when you needed assistance or wanted to be transported to camp. The video also discussed route signage, gear handling, tent assignment and etiquette, camp dining hours, and the sink and shower trucks. Lastly, it mentioned the special tents in camp: Camp Services, event headquarters; Medical Services, which included a self-help area; the 3-Day Store; the 3-Day Café, where there were inflatable couches, magazines, decks of cards, and toenail polish; and, off by itself, the Remembrance Tent.

In 2004, we watched the safety video prior to check-in on what was called "Day 0," which was the Thursday before the first day of the walk on Friday (Day 1). This procedure was computerized for 2005, eliminating Day 0. In 2004, after watching the video and signing a participant waiver, we checked in, turned in medical history forms and any remaining donations, purchased towel service for $10 (optional, but highly recommended), and received our tent assignments. We were then issued our official 3-Day credentials, which we wore around our necks in a plastic sleeve on a lanyard. The plastic sleeve also provided a place to keep our daily route cards and a flat surface for the stickers that we would receive during the next three days.

The last time that I was as excited about being rewarded with stickers was when I was seven years old and taking piano lessons. Back then, the stickers were either foil stars or a little black piano on an orange background. The latter was only awarded when the assignment was mastered, which was, for me, after a succession of hopeful stars. By the time I finally learned the piece, the music sheet was pretty much used up by stickers. Forty-five years later, by the time I finished the 3-Day, the plastic sleeve of my credential was, similarly, pretty much used up by stickers that had been given out along the route. The people who gave us the stickers were mainly members of the various 3-Day volunteer crews but, in some cases, friends and family members at cheering stations passed them out.

Sometimes the stickers coincided with the theme of the Pit Stop or the Grab & Go stations. These rest stops were located every two or three miles along the route and had booths with water and Gatorade® and porta-potties. The Pit Stops had snacks and medical assistance. These stations also provided entertainment. The volunteer crews who staffed these rest stops seemed to be competing to see who could come up with the cleverest theme. They went all out: costumes, decorations, music, stickers (of course), and sometimes even little souvenirs like beads and pins and bracelets. People along the route also gave us things. One man and his two young children dressed up like pirates. They were along the route all three days, playing pirate music and doling out gold-coin chocolate pieces from a treasure chest.

AOL® for Broadband, Motrin®, and New Balance®—major sponsors for the 2004 3-Day events—also had Pit Stops. They gave us socks, headbands, sunscreen, blinking lights, and, to add to our collections of plastic beads, lip balm on a string. Between Friday morning (Day 1) when we left Topsfield Fairgrounds and Sunday afternoon (Day 3) when we circled Bunker Hill Monument and arrived to cheering friends and family members at Bunker Hill Community College, we had been given so much gaudy stuff to drape, pin, clip, and stick on ourselves that we looked like we had been partying at Mardi Gras.

At a Pit Stop on Day 3, one of the volunteers, seeing that I was wearing a pink survivor's cap, asked me, "You're a survivor, right?" When I said yes, he gave me a white ceramic angel pin with the pink ribbon emblem on her dress, holding a pink heart above her head. It was affixed to a presentation card that read, "Heart of a Survivor." He explained that as he and the other volunteers were setting up the Pit Stop, a woman, who was backing out of her driveway at a nearby house, lowered her car window and asked him what they were doing. When he told her, she pulled forward into her driveway, went inside the house, and returned with the pin. She told the volunteer that she couldn't stay to do so herself, but asked him if he would give the pin to a breast cancer survivor. When the volunteer told me the story, he got tears in his eyes. Without hesitation, I wrapped my arms around this stranger and hugged him. Tears came to my eyes as well.

For many participants, hugging is as integral to the 3-Day as walking. So is being nice, helpful, and emotionally open. This phenomenon was summarized at Opening Ceremonies by Howard Sitron, who was then the National Philanthropic Trust's vice president and chief operating officer of the 3-Day, when he promised, "For the next three days, the world will be the way you have always wanted it to be." Truth told, when Howard Sitron said that, I was skeptical.

Writing about hugging, being nice, and being helpful would have rung my hokey bell before participating in the 3-Day events. If described at all, I would have used side glances and metaphors to scrub away all the spontaneity. Even reading about these interactions was too soupy for me. That kind of sentimentality seemed contrived. However, as I was to learn, participating in the 3-Day was an opportunity for many people to pause long enough for valid emotions to catch up. The irony of walking 60 miles as a way to be still is inescapable, of course.

Before the 3-Day, my grief for the recent deaths of my father and my husband was often "tamped down," as I called it. To avoid crying, I actually made downward-sweeping hand motions like I was quieting applause—my physical way to reinforce the tamping down of emotions. I eventually discovered, though, that one of the toxic side effects of compartmentalizing sadness was the blunting of all emotions, including positive ones, like creativity and enthusiasm and joy. It was my trade-off for appearing strong. When I thought about it, I even imagined a shiny steel ball in my forehead, full of tears that I would never release. Until the 3-Day, I hid my sadness, as did another woman whom I met on my way back to my tent after dinner on Day 2.

The sleeping tents were on the fenced soccer field at Beverly High School. The big dining tent and the other smaller, special tents were on an adjacent sweep of grass next to the high school auditorium. To get from one area to the next, we passed through a gate with a pole sticking up in the middle, which was probably there to prevent people from riding motorcycles back and forth; however, it also meant that only one person at a time could pass through the gate.

As I approached the gate from one direction, Geralyn McPhail was approaching from the other. I noticed her because she looked surprisingly fresh and rested for someone who had just walked 20 miles. She had long, brown hair and was wearing a camisole t-shirt that revealed feminine but sturdy shoulders and upper arms. I later learned that she was 47 years old; however, she looked much younger. She motioned for me to go ahead of her and, when I said thanks, we made eye contact. In a New England accent, she said, smiling broadly, "Isn't this event great?"

"Oh, yes," I replied. "This has been one of the most meaningful experiences I've ever had."

Without warning, the smile faded, her chin quivered, and she started to cry. "I'm sorry," she said. "I don't know why I'm crying so much. I've been crying off and on since yesterday at Opening Ceremonies." Motioning toward my cap, she said, "You're a survivor. So's my little sister and my mother."

I touched her arm and said, "How long has your sister been a survivor?"

"She was diagnosed in 2003, so in May, it was a year since she was diagnosed, only she'd had it for 11 months before that but her doctors didn't do anything about it. They just kept telling her that they'd keep an eye on it and to come back in six months. By the time it was diagnosed, the tumor was something like 3 cm, and there was a microscopic spot of cancer in one of the lymph nodes."

Geralyn McPhail's sister, Norma Logan, was 45 years old when her gynecologist referred her for a screening mammogram. Their mother had been diagnosed with breast cancer at age 50, so the sisters were at a mildly increased risk for developing breast cancer. Although Norma's clinical breast exam by the gynecologist was negative, the mammogram showed a mass. The gynecologist suggested that Norma wait another six months and repeat the mammogram. However, about a month after the mammogram, Norma was able to feel the mass and made an appointment with a local surgeon. He, too, didn't think there was anything to worry about and suggested a conservative, wait-and-see approach.

Since the surgeon was considered to be the best one in their area of Connecticut, Norma was reassured by his opinion that the mass was benign, and she didn't pursue the matter beyond this point; however, her agreement to delay further diagnostic procedures was far from a wide-eyed innocent's acceptance of a doctor's recommendation. Norma had worked in the medical and pharmaceutical industry for over 25 years, including a 10-year stint doing breast cancer research for Fred Hutchinson Cancer Research Center in Seattle, Washington.

Unfortunately, Norma's follow-up mammogram showed progression of the mass that was being followed as well as suspicious calcifications in the opposite breast. A needle biopsy of the mass was positive for invasive cancer.

Geralyn described how she learned about her sister's diagnosis: "She got the diagnosis on Friday afternoon and called me on Saturday morning. I told her, 'I'm coming right over.' I grabbed my boyfriend and went to her house. I knew I had to be strong for her. She's so little—no bigger than a peanut. She cried. We all cried. I told her, 'You have the biggest fight of your life ahead of you.' My sister doesn't come to me for advice, but she comes to me because she knows that I will have the most honest reaction, and she knows I'll always be there for her.

"When I left my sister that day, she was going to be calling my mom. I told her to give me enough time to get to Ma's house, so I can be there for her. I knew my mom was going to be upset. When I got there, Ma kept saying how guilty she felt that she'd given Norma breast cancer. I told her that, 'Yeah, it can be genetic, but it happens. It just happens.' Still, she felt so guilty. I kept wondering why it had to be her [Norma], because she was the little one. I didn't have any answers, so I was at the computer trying to get information."

Geralyn was accustomed to solving problems. She worked as a cable splicer for Southwestern Bell Communications and had been with the company for 25 years. When I asked her what a cable splicer does, she said, "I work on the poles, in the manholes, on the circuits." With a chuckle, she added, "I put it all together to make it work."

That explained why Geralyn looked so sturdy and strong. Still, for someone who had worked outside for decades, she had a beautiful complexion. Also, her mannerisms and speech were surprisingly delicate for a woman who spent her days doing physically demanding work among men. About her career choice, she said, "At first, I worked in the office, but as soon as I could, I went outside. That's where I like it the best. Besides, I was a single mom for a long time and the money was good. My dad was a lineman for the power company, and I used to ride around in the truck with him. I always enjoyed doing that."

After Norma learned that she had cancer, she sought a second opinion from a medical oncologist at New York University. She ultimately decided to be treated in her Connecticut hometown. This consisted of bilateral mastectomy and removal of the axillary lymph nodes on the side with invasive cancer, followed by eight courses of adjuvant chemotherapy and full-course radiation. She did not receive adjuvant hormonal therapy because her tumor was estrogen-receptor (ER) negative. She also decided against reconstructive surgery.

Norma's husband had no objection to her decision to forego reconstructive surgery. About her brother-in-law, Geralyn said, "He's a really great guy. They don't have any children, so they are very close. When she was having treatment, I offered to help, but he was with her every step of the way. I would have loved to have been able to do more. I weeded her garden for her. I really wanted to do more, but they had it under control, which was the best way for them."

In contrast to Norma (who was angry at *herself* for not having a diagnostic procedure done earlier), Geralyn directed her anger at the doctors for their part in delaying diagnosis. This emotion was mixed with fear and sadness that her sister might not survive the cancer. She was also frustrated that she couldn't do more to help her sister. Her usual take-charge way of doing things—putting it all together and making it work—was worthless when it came to her sister's breast cancer. The only contribution she hoped to make was to appear strong for her sister and her mother. Consequently, she kept her feelings inside—that is, until the Boston 3-Day.

During our conversation, she intermittently became tearful. And, when she told me a story about an angel charm, I became tearful as well. One morning, when Geralyn was filling up her work truck with gas, she and a stranger struck up a conversation. Before he left, he reached over between the gas pumps and handed her an inexpensive, gold-painted angel on a chain. When she climbed back into her truck, she tied the angel on the vent. From then on, every time she started to worry about her sister, she held the little angel and said a prayer.

"I prayed for my sister all the time because she's my little angel. It was like one of those worry stones. Even after I rubbed off all the paint, I still held on to it and prayed for my sister. I do a lot of driving, so my mind was always going to her during the day, and that angel was something to hold on to. It kept me sane. I'd think of my sister and reach for the angel. After the chain broke, I carried the angel in my wallet. I was always praying for my sister. Me, I'm much more outgoing and aggressive. She's such a private person and with her, it's easier not to talk. I don't know if she knows how much I love her. When she got cancer, it made me realize how much I love her."

About five months after the Boston 3-Day, I called Geralyn to clarify some of the details of our conversation. I asked her what, in retrospect, had been the best part of the 3-Day for her. At first, she talked about everyone's kindness and how inspirational it was that everyone was there for the same reason. Her voice softened and she said, "Until that walk, I felt like I had to be strong all the time. But there, I got to spend three days with my sister, and I could finally let go because she was next to me being strong."

———————

That evening, before lights out, the Men With Heart comedy team was at it again:

"No more conversations about your panties tonight, okay?"

"I'm not wearing panties."

(mumble, mumble)

"What's that noise?"

"It's my zipper."

(mumble, mumble)

"Oh, don't touch me there."

(mumble, mumble)

"People are going to wonder why our tent is shaking."

"We can tell them it's the wind."

"Nah, they're too smart for that."

"Oh, yeah. I forgot. They're women."

Later that night, when everything was quiet, I pulled back the tent flap and looked at the sky. Overhead, the second full moon that month— a "Blue Moon"—was in a clear space, completely surrounded by clouds. The moon was back-illuminating the clouds, creating a bright circle around it. I lay there in the quiet, knowing that I was surrounded by over a thousand people, all with stories, all with their own reasons for being there.

Some were there because, like Geralyn McPhail, they had felt so helpless against a disease that threatened someone they loved. Like Geralyn, they had been fearful that their loved one's cancer might not completely respond to surgery, chemotherapy, and radiation. Like Geralyn, they were terrified that the cancer might recur. I had been in both situations, and I knew that it was easier to be a cancer patient than it was to helplessly watch as two people whom I loved suffer and die. I looked at the bright circle around that big Blue Moon, and I didn't even try to tamp down the tears.

As I was waiting in line the next morning to brush my teeth, I met Robbie Lacritz Deitch, a petite woman with shoulder-length brown hair, wearing a pink survivor's cap. We talked about how much fun we were having and how we hoped that we could finish the day's walk without having to be "swept" by bus or van to Closing Ceremonies. She asked me how long it had been since I finished chemotherapy, and I told her that I had been treated with wide local excision and radiation but no chemotherapy. Sensing that she must have had chemotherapy, I told her how pretty her hair was. She smiled slyly and said, "Oh, this isn't my real hair." She pulled up the edge of her cap to show that her hair was really a hula skirt-like wig.

I told her that my fiancé was a medical oncologist and that he thought "chemo hair" (the first regrowth of hair after treatment-induced hair loss) was the most beautiful hair he had ever seen. Robbie yanked off her cap, revealing a quarter-inch of new growth, and, like it was a wicked secret, she whispered, "I *love* my new hair." I gently touched her lamb's fuzz and kissed her on the top her head. We laughed and hugged each other. I later asked her to share her story.

Robbie was 54 years old and, until her 50th birthday, she worked as a clinical psychologist. Following retirement, she became a self-described "volunteer queen." Eight months before the Boston 3-Day— right after Robbie and her family returned from a winter vacation to Rio de Janeiro—she noticed that she had a "weird sort of cold." Since there had been a lot of "partying and drinking and kissing," she figured that she had contracted an unusual virus in South America. She took the usual over-the-counter medicines to treat her symptoms; however, there was still no improvement after two weeks. In fact, she was getting worse. Her breathing had become so labored that she could no longer swim her morning laps. She visited her primary care physician who, after listening to her chest with a stethoscope, said that it sounded like she had bronchitis. He prescribed antibiotics and told her that he would order an x-ray if there was no improvement over the next five days.

By the time she had the chest x-ray the following Monday, Robbie's difficult breathing had progressed to the point that she couldn't climb a flight of stairs. The chest x-ray showed "fluid around the lungs," so Robbie was referred to a pulmonologist (a lung doctor). First, she ordered an echocardiogram (an imaging study of the heart) to rule out heart failure as the underlying cause of the fluid accumulation in the chest cavity. That study was normal. In fact, it showed that Robbie's heart was "performing like that of a 35-year-old athlete." She scheduled a CAT [computerized axial tomography] scan for the following Monday.

That weekend, she and her sister made a quick trip to Florida. Robbie remembered being in a bad mood the whole weekend, griping about her doctor. She was convinced that he had prescribed the wrong antibiotics for the unusual South American bug to which she thought she'd been exposed.

Robbie was a cheerful, friendly woman. I had trouble picturing her in a grumpy mood. I suspected that, since her lungs couldn't expand because of the fluid, her bad mood had been due to hypoxia (air hunger). I knew about hypoxia. During two of my four bouts of radiation pneumonitis (lung inflammation), hypoxia brought forth a less-than-charming side to my personality. As my hypoxia resolved, so did my bitchiness— or, to be more precise, it returned to baseline.

The day after she returned from Florida, Robbie underwent a CAT scan, which, like the chest x-ray, was normal except for the chest cavity fluid. The radiologist described the amount of fluid as being "like the first three stories of a five-story building being underwater." Two days later, she had a procedure to remove the fluid but, by then, she couldn't lie down to sleep. The pulmonologist tapped nearly a liter of fluid from one lung cavity. Robbie was immediately able to breathe more easily but was surprised when she saw that the fluid that had been removed was "pinky-red instead of clear," as she had assumed it would be. She concluded, "I must have a blood clot." The fluid was sent to Pathology for evaluation.

The following day, her pulmonologist phoned and asked her to come to her office. She added, "And bring someone with you." Robbie and her friend, Carol, were planning to have lunch and go shopping that day, so Robbie asked Carol if she would mind going along with her to the pulmonologist's office.

Robbie also called her husband at work who said, "I'm on my way." Robbie told him that it wasn't necessary for him to leave work since Carol was going with her, but he repeated, "I'm on my way."

Robbie, her husband, and Carol were sitting together in the pulmonologist's office when they learned that the microscopic examination of the fluid from the chest cavity had shown tumor cells that were most likely derived from metastatic ovarian cancer. This meant that Robbie had Stage IV disease. The first question that she asked the pulmonologist was, "There's a Stage V, right?" When she heard the negative answer, her first thought was, You are not talking about me. I have this shield. No way this is about me.

Her second thought was about 20 cases of wine that she had recently purchased. "Right before my diagnosis, I had bought some wine by e-mail—a promotional thing where we buy our wine. When I went to pick it up, I realized there were 20 cases of wine. I thought, Oh, my gosh, what will my husband say? He'll think I've gone crazy buying all this wine. So my friend and I snuck it into our wine cellar. When I got the diagnosis, all I could think about was that some of that wine needed to be in the cellar for 10 years. I thought, I'm not going anywhere until every last bottle of that wine is gone."

After she learned the diagnosis, she immediately called a medical oncologist, who was a long-time friend. "When I met my husband, Jeff and I were dating. He was an oncology resident at the time. While he was never meant to be the man I married, we have remained friends throughout the years, mainly because I have a lot of cancer in my family. He treated my father for Hodgkin's disease and both my mother and my sister for breast cancer. My sister was diagnosed at age 30 and has had three recurrences. She's fine now. Jeff treated me like I was his wife. I went directly from the pulmonologist's office to his. Over the next two days, I had CAT scans and MRIs [magnetic resonance imaging] and pelvic ultrasounds, which were all negative, but the CA 125 was very elevated."

Although CA 125 (a blood test) can be elevated for a number of benign reasons, in Robbie's case it was because of metastatic cancer. CA 125 is the most reliable serum tumor marker for investigating ovarian cancer. If a woman has an abnormal pelvic mass and an elevated CA 125, there is about a 90% chance that the mass is malignant. In addition to being helpful for establishing the diagnosis of ovarian cancer, CA 125 can also be useful for predicting the length of survival (determining prognosis or predicted outcome), for gauging the response to treatment, and for detecting a relapse (recurrence). In fact, serial determinations of CA 125 are a sensitive and specific way to monitor a patient for recurrence after surgery.

Robbie's tests were soon complete and the presumptive diagnosis was metastatic ovarian cancer. Further studies were planned; however, within three days, Robbie called her medical oncologist and told him that she was losing a pound a day and wanted to start chemotherapy immediately. Her friend agreed and, within two days—almost exactly a month after she first saw her primary care physician for what she thought was a cold—she started the first of six rounds of paclitaxel (Taxol®) and carboplatin (Paraplatin®).

Robbie lost her thick, shoulder-length dark hair after the first course of chemotherapy. She bought four wigs, including the one that she was wearing when I met her—the one she called her "athletic wig." She had also worn this wig when she trained for the 3-Day. She said that anticipating the Boston 3-Day was an anchor for her during chemotherapy. "Right through the treatments, I had this vision of walking over the finish line in my pink shirt. I kept visualizing that. I wanted to be able to say, 'Yeah, I did that.'"

That afternoon at Bunker Hill Community College, as we participants waited in the holding area for Closing Ceremonies to start, I spotted Robbie in the pink survivor's t-shirt that she had received at the end of the walk. She was surrounded by a group of people who I later learned were her husband, her mother, her 18-year-old son, her son's former babysitter (who Robbie described as being "like my older son") and his girlfriend, her niece, and her niece's college roommate. Robbie was radiant, laughing, energetic, and obviously joyful. She wasn't wearing her cap and the wig dangled from her wrist.

Based on serial evaluations of CA 125, Robbie Deitch achieved a short remission. She was in remission when she participated in the Boston 3-Day; however, I talked to Robbie again in November 2004, and her CA 125 had begun to climb again. This was a grave sign that signaled tumor recurrence. She said, "At some point, it sinks in, but I remind myself that any one of us can walk out the door and get hit by a truck. *Anything* can happen when you walk out there. The thing with cancer is that there is some control. At least with cancer, someone is paying attention. Also, I meet all four criteria for people who do well with cancer—spirituality, basic good health, a support system, and a positive attitude. I figure I have great odds. Besides, I live in Boston. The best treatment available anywhere is available to me. Every year that they keep me alive, it's that much more likely that they'll find something else that works to keep me going."

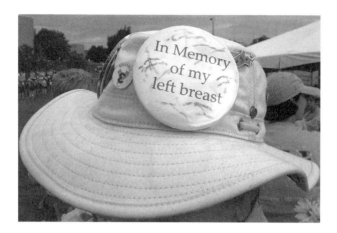

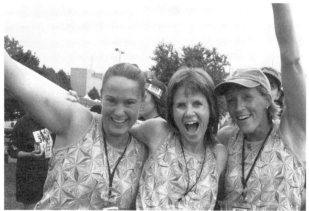

Loree McCary, DawnElla Rust and Jennie Collings

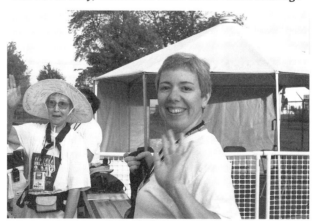

Jennifer Stewart

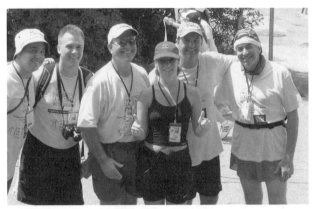

Men With Heart

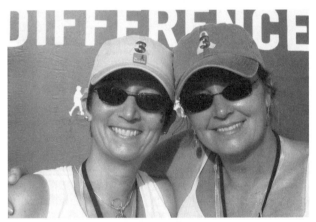

Sisters Norma Logan and Geralyn McPhail

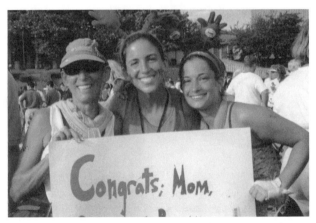

Robbie Lacritz Deitch, far left, with team members

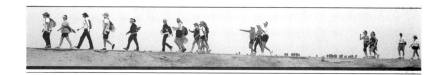

Chapter 2

New York
August 6, August 7, and August 8, 2004

As I waited in the security checkpoint line at the San Antonio International Airport, I watched a Transportation Security Administration (TSA) inspector view the x-ray images of carry-on items as they passed through the scanner. She peered at her computer screen, leaning slightly forward at the waist, back rigid, blue-gloved hands poised at the keyboard. Periodically, she leaned closer to the screen, chin jutted, and squinted at something, fingers twitching on the keys. She continued to stare as she straightened up, cocked her head, and laced her fingers together as if she were about to play the children's hand motion rhyme, "Here's the church, here's the steeple." The carry-on item either advanced along the conveyor belt or she motioned for a manual inspection.

All TSA personnel have important assignments, but the job of deciphering a mishmash of multicolored shapes seems particularly crucial. Furthermore, the subjectivity of interpreting mishmash must add to the stress. The longer I watched, the more curious I became about what, exactly, triggered a manual inspection. I thought better of asking about it—security measures being what they were—because I didn't want my name to end up on some list. (In fact, I want this written down for everyone to see: I don't care one whit about shapes or colors or any of that stuff. No, sirree, not one whit.)

Okay. So.

Parallels exist between a TSA inspector looking for suspicious shapes on a computer screen and a surgical pathologist looking for breast cancer on a microscope slide. Both are searching for something that they do not want to find and, based on *subjective* visual cues, must decide if what they are looking at is a threat. For the TSA official, the lives of hundreds, or even thousands, of people may be at risk; for the surgical pathologist, it is the health of one patient. In both cases, though, a moment's inattention could have grave consequences. I cannot fathom the degree of stress that a TSA official endures; however, I know about that kind of stress from the personal experience of a surgical pathologist.

Until I retired from the practice of pathology in 2002, evaluation of breast biopsies always caused me to sit up straight with my jaw clenched and anal sphincter tight. This was particularly so during the early years of my career when one-stage surgical procedures for breast cancer were still the standard of care in our part of the country. This meant that the surgeon sent the breast biopsy tissue to the pathologist for a rapid diagnosis using frozen section technique while the patient was still under anesthesia. If the pathologist's diagnosis was benign (noncancerous), the surgeon closed the patient's incision and sent her to the Recovery Room; if malignant (cancerous), the surgeon would usually do a modified radical mastectomy on the affected side, which involved removal of the entire breast, with nipple, areola, and surrounding skin, plus removal of all axillary (armpit) lymph nodes. Breast conservation surgery, which I will talk about later, did not become common practice in our part of the country until I had been in practice for about 15 years.

A "false positive" on frozen section—meaning that the pathologist interpreted the slide as cancer, but it turned out the following day to be benign on permanent (or "final") sections—was unforgivable, since this meant that the patient had undergone an unnecessary mastectomy. A "false negative" on frozen section—meaning the pathologist missed the cancer on frozen section but found it on final sections—was not as calamitous, of course, but it was still frowned upon, since the preferred one-stage procedure would, necessarily, become a two-stage procedure: a diagnostic biopsy first; a therapeutic mastectomy later. Furthermore— and this is not trivial—a "false negative" discrepancy created an emotional seesaw for the patient who was initially reassured by the surgeon, based on the frozen section results, that everything was okay, but later learned that cancer was there, after all, and further surgery was necessary.

Since the surgeon and his or her assistants are—quite literally— standing around and waiting for the results of the frozen section, the pathologist does not dawdle. In fact, the faster, the better. Usually, but not always, the pathologist knows that a frozen section is scheduled and stays in or near the lab to avoid wasting precious minutes while hurrying back from the cafeteria or the doctors' lounge.

The biopsy tissue is delivered to the lab by someone from the Operating Room or arrives via chute. First, the pathologist does a gross exam of the tissue (described in Chapter 1). If a specimen radiograph accompanies the biopsy, it is used to pinpoint the suspicious area. Based primarily on the tissue's appearance and consistency, a piece of tissue that is about a square centimeter is selected for the actual frozen section examination. (Tick. Tick. Tick.)

The tissue cube is transferred to a brass "button," slathered with gooey mounting medium, and placed on a freezing tray in a subzero box called a cryostat, which is outfitted with a blade for thinly slicing tissue. The brass button, with its precious cargo of frozen tissue, is then fastened to a platform and advanced toward the blade by means of the cryostat control panel. At first, the cryostat operator (the pathologist or the technician) advances the tissue relatively rapidly, but as the precious (and irreplaceable) part of the tissue approaches the blade, the operator decelerates advancement so that the tissue won't be inadvertently shaved away. (If this occurs, the tissue is, for all intents and purposes, lost forever.)

As the tissue is rapidly advancing toward the blade, the slices are about as thick as tissue paper and are composed mainly of frozen mounting medium. As the diagnostic part of the tissue surfaces, the cryostat operator adjusts the advancement mechanism so that the slices are as thin as spider webs. When a complete cross section of the tissue is achieved, this slice (or "level") is wicked onto a glass slide. (Tick. Tick. Tick.)

The tissue level is virtually transparent and must be stained by sequentially dipping the slide in special dyes, various alcohol concentrations, and a clearing agent, such as xylene. After staining, the slide is cover-glassed and ready for the pathologist to look at under the microscope. If all has gone swimmingly, the pathologist has a thin, well-stained microscopic section of the suspicious area, and he or she calmly—without interruptions or distractions—interprets the pink and purple mishmash under the microscope, renders a diagnosis, and reports the findings to the surgeon. Again, if all has gone swimmingly. Yeah, right ...

Sometimes, another frozen section examination, from another surgical procedure, is underway, and the breast biopsy has to wait its turn. This happens more often when the pathologist works alone at a small hospital, which was the situation for much of my career. Sometimes, more than one suspicious area is identified by gross examination and two or three—not just one—sections are needed. For mysterious reasons, the frozen tissue sometimes decides to pop off the surface of the brass button during sectioning, or the spider web-like section folds in half or floats off the slide during the staining steps (*damn it!*). Sometimes, a nitwit (that would be me) leaves the cryostat door a tiny bit ajar, the temperature of the freezing tray rises, and the freezing process is prolonged (*damn it!*). Sometimes, additional ("deeper") levels are required to confirm the diagnosis or, in the thick of things, the phone rings and the principal at your son's school insists on speaking to you. Immediately ... (Tick.Tick.Tick.)

Eventualities like these cost precious ticks and, believe me, if the diagnosis is delayed, the Operating Room is calling on the phone, or the intercom, or both, and asking, *"What's the holdup?"* Honestly, though, can you blame them?

When I was doing a frozen section and realized that I couldn't have a diagnosis within 15 minutes, I always let the surgeon know. In most instances, Morris, or Jeff, or Boyce, or Skeet, or John E. would say, "No problem, Debbey. Take your time." (God, I loved those men—every one of them.)

When a patient's breast was in the balance, I was always grateful for the relatively straightforward diagnoses and scared strawless by the tough cases—the "hard calls." Fortunately, two-stage procedures replaced one-stage procedures as the standard of care for breast lesions in the early 1990s. Nowadays, a diagnostic procedure is done first—most often a core biopsy, a fine-needle aspiration biopsy, or, less often, an open surgical biopsy—and a therapeutic surgical procedure is done later. Another major shift from the old days, of course, is that patients are involved with treatment decisions.

As new tests were developed, the way in which biopsy tissue was handled evolved, too. For instance, estrogen- and progesterone-receptor status determines whether adjuvant hormonal treatment will benefit the patient, and freezing breast lesions confounds the ultimate interpretation of those results. When determination of receptor status became the standard of care, pathologists were off the hook for doing frozen sections on breast lesions that were less than a centimeter.

———

As I waited in line at the airport to leave for New York on that August morning, TSA officials were definitely not off the hook. Three days before, Homeland Security Secretary Tom Ridge had raised the terror alert level to Code Orange—the second highest level on the government's five-level scale—for the financial services sectors of northern New Jersey; Washington, D.C.; and New York City. This warning resulted from the discovery of new plans of attack on the United States and Britain after the capture of Ahmed Khalfan Ghailani, a high-ranking al-Qaida operative. A confiscated computer contained detailed surveillance information on five key financial sites. The sophistication of the information was unusual, describing the best places for reconnaissance, how to make contact with employees who work in the buildings, traffic patterns, and security details.

Although the new intelligence seemed to indicate that the terrorists would prefer to use car or truck bombs, TSA officials remained sharp-eyed for that needle (or other potential weapon) in the stacks and stacks of carry-on items. As Morris and the other surgeons had done for me when I was doing frozen sections, I wanted to assure the TSA inspector that I didn't mind waiting. "Just take your time," I wanted to say. "If you must, lean close for every color jumble. Please, do what is necessary to be absolutely sure."

———

About a thousand walkers and 200 volunteer crew members participated in the New York 3-Day event. Of the 10 2004 Breast Cancer 3-Day events, New York's would turn out to have the fewest number of participants. I overheard an event organizer say that 800 people who had preregistered and forwarded donations to the Susan G. Komen Foundation did not show up. The Orange Alert was blamed for this.

Howard Sitron, who was then the National Philanthropic Trust vice president and chief operating officer of the Breast Cancer 3-Day, alluded to the situation during Opening Ceremonies when he said, "Recent news has kept some walkers at home." His tone was not the least bit reproachful. Among those who walked, despite concerns, was Cheryl Rogers.

Cheryl was a Hollywood screen actor who lived in Brooklyn and worked for New York Public Radio as assistant to Laura Walker, the president and chief executive officer of WNYC radio. Cheryl previously worked for *Ms. Magazine* and was on her way to work at their offices in Manhattan on September 11, 2001. The first tower had collapsed just moments before she got off the subway and, instead of going to work, she joined the thousands of people who were fleeing the smoke. As she crossed the Brooklyn Bridge, she heard "a bunch of snapping sounds" and turned to watch in horror as the second tower collapsed. "We were all crying. It was as if the two towers just disappeared. I don't think anyone thought about them collapsing—maybe burned-out shells of buildings, but not collapsing. All I could think about was that I wanted to get home. I wanted to find out if a friend who worked across the street from where I did was okay. I wanted to let my family know that I was okay, but I wanted to get home. I wanted to get home and feed my cat. I stayed in my apartment and cried for five days. It was such an invasive thing—slamming planes into buildings. After 9/11, I was paralyzed with fear."

Cheryl told me her story within 15 minutes of our first meeting. She, Linda Jackson (the breast cancer survivor whom I was interviewing), and I were eating lunch at Corona Park in Queens on Day 1 of the walk. As we sat cross-legged on the grass, airplanes roared overhead every three minutes, headed toward John F. Kennedy International Airport. We chatted about how glad we were that the weather had warmed up from that morning's 62 degrees; we talked about what we were having for lunch (chicken sandwiches, chips, an apple, big chewy cookies); we marveled at the variety and abundance of cellophane-packaged snacks at the Pit Stops. Linda, who was walking in her fourth 3-Day event, commented on the relatively small number of walkers who were participating in 2004, which, she said, contrasted with previous years when several thousand people had participated. This led to Cheryl's story about 9/11.

The language and tone of Cheryl's story suggested that she had told it many times. I had had a similar impression two days before—the almost compulsive need to share a story—when the Armenian American cabdriver, unbidden, talked about 9/11. He had seen the second plane hit the World Trade Center and had watched as people jumped from the towers. His voice thickened when he said, "I cried like a baby. Just like a baby." I didn't know what to say to him, and I tried to avert my eyes from his big shoulders rocking and the tears trickling down his cheek.

During the New York 3-Day, I heard (and overheard) other recitations of 9/11 experiences. Almost every time, the stories sounded as if they had been told many times before. That made me consider why someone would repeat a story so often that it sounded as if they had learned it by rote. Maybe they hoped that the retelling would dilute the horror, or give it some meaning, or contain their feelings, or even achieve some sense of community. Maybe they imagined that if they said it out loud something magical would happen—that the listener would say, "You must be imagining things. That never happened." Or, maybe they were bearing witness for those who will never speak again.

When people shared their cancer stories during the 3-Day events, their voices, like those of the 9/11 storytellers, often verged on singsong. The stories and the storytellers' ultimate goals were different, though. First of all, the cancer stories were not historical in the sense that the 9/11 stories were historical; they were personal. Secondly, among other reasons for sharing their cancer stories, I sensed that many also saw it as a way to *help* the listener. It wasn't until the Arizona 3-Day—the last event in 2004—did anyone say it directly, though.

But I'm getting way ahead of myself.

———

Cheryl Rogers and Linda Jackson, 51, had been friends since 1986, when they met at Chautauqua Institution, which is a summer arts festival in the southwestern corner of New York State. Chautauqua has its own dance, theater, and opera companies, and its own symphony orchestra. When they met, Cheryl had been hired as an actor by Michael Kahn, and Linda was the managing director of the opera company. The theater and opera companies sometimes collaborated on productions, and the two women became friends. They worked together for only three summers at Chautauqua but have remained friends. They periodically meet in "the city" for a show or drinks, and sometimes go dancing at the Culture Club if, as Cheryl said, they "need to work out something that's not right."

Linda added, "We used to go dancing a lot. We would be the oldest people in the place, but it didn't matter, because dancing was just a necessary thing. Just *dancing*."

Linda's first 3-Day event was in September 2000, just four months after she had undergone a bilateral mastectomy with reconstructive surgery following the diagnosis of her second breast cancer episode. She was first diagnosed with breast cancer in 1999, when she was 46 years old. Although no mass was palpable, her annual screening mammogram showed two areas of suspicious calcification, which were core-biopsied and found to be benign; however, in another area of her breast, away from the calcifications, cancer was discovered.

When asked if the diagnosis frightened her, she shook her head and shrugged. "No, not really. I figured if you're sick, you go to the doctor and they fix it; then you're not sick anymore. The only thing that scared me was the anesthesia. I wasn't afraid of dying, but I just didn't want to end up in a coma. Before I had the mastectomies, I sometimes thought about recurrence. I once asked my doctor how I would know if I was going to get cancer in another part of my body. His answer was, 'You don't.'"

Linda described a friend who wasn't feeling well, went to the doctor, and learned that he had widely metastatic disease. She said, "Cancer is like a terrorist attack. You can't do much to prevent it."

As she considered treatment options for her first breast cancer, Linda called seven friends who were breast cancer survivors and whose ages at diagnosis were between 25 and 68 years old. "Some of them had radiation; some had chemo; some had lumpectomies; some had mastectomies; some had reconstruction. I called them so that I could ask them what to expect—what would happen—and they were great. It was as if I were now part of a group."

As she talked with more and more friends about their breast cancer diagnoses and treatments, Linda developed another emotion in addition to gratitude. "I somehow knew all along that I would get cancer—although there was no logical reason to think that—so I wasn't angry about my own diagnosis. On one hand, I was glad that I had friends whom I could talk to but, on the other hand, I was angry that there were *so many* people I knew who had cancer."

Actually, it's not surprising that Linda knew seven women with breast cancer, since a woman has a one in seven lifetime risk of being diagnosed with cancer. Considering the hundreds of people whom she has met during her career, it was actually surprising that she didn't know even more women to call.

And what a career! I found the following biography on the Internet:

Linda Jackson ... is the Managing Director of Connecticut Opera, having previously served as the General Director of the Berkshire Opera Company since August 2001. From 1998 until moving to the Berkshires she served as the Executive Director for the Byrd Hoffman Foundation, and during the 1997-1998 season she worked as the Artistic Administrator for Opera Pacific. In 1997, Linda traveled to 63 U.S. cities as the Company Manager for the New York City Opera National Company production of La Boheme, *and from 1994-1996 she was the General Manager for 651, an Arts Center at the Brooklyn Academy of Music. Linda spent 1981 through 1994 at the Chautauqua Opera in the following capacities: Production Stage Manager (1981-1982), Production Manager (1983-1984), Managing Director (1985-1987), and finally General Director (1988-1994). From 1984-1987 she served as Production Manager for Texas Opera Theater—the touring arm of Houston Grand Opera, was the Production Stage Manager for Greater Miami Opera from 1981-1984, and was the Stage Manager for Houston Grand Opera from 1977-1980. Prior to beginning her career in Opera, Linda worked with several Off-Off Broadway companies including Jean Erdman's Theater of the Open Eye. She holds a degree in English and Theater Arts from Douglass College.*

(During several hours of conversation at the New York 3-Day, she occasionally alluded to these activities, but *my word*. I had no idea about her accomplishments until I was doing some Internet sleuthing about Chautauqua and decided to search "Linda Jackson opera." No wonder I felt intimidated when we were walking together, despite her friendliness and sense of humor. I had assumed that it was because she was taller than I was.)

When Linda was a college freshman, she considered studying law or going to seminary. Her dorm was across the quadrangle from the college's theater and "on a lark," she stopped by the theater office and offered to help build scenery. (In high school, she had built scenery for the school plays and had enjoyed it.) The man behind the desk happened to be the instructor for Theater Basics 101 Craft Design and suggested that, instead of volunteering backstage, she sign up for his class. She agreed, since she needed an elective anyway, and started working backstage on shows. By her junior year, she had decided to combine a theater major with her English major.

This decision coincided with her increasing disillusionment with the Presbyterian church that she attended. This change of heart took place during the early 1970s, when she could not square being a Christian and supporting the Vietnam War. Also, the liberal, progressive minister with whom she had grown up had supported social outreach programs; he was replaced by another pastor who focused on the gospel at the expense of community activities. Lastly, her father, a retired New York State Supreme Court judge, after years of asking her why she didn't go to law school, finally validated her dream when he said, after seeing one of her shows, "You know, Linda, you are really good at this. You could do it for a living."

So instead of law school or seminary, she applied to graduate school at New York University in theater, where she studied for a year. Classroom studies were soon replaced by real-world challenges when a professor, who was producing a show Off-Broadway, asked her to stage-manage for him. Through this opportunity, she met other people in the business and eventually started freelancing as a stage manager in New York. It wasn't long before a man whom she had met in college asked her if she would assist him with an opera production. She loved it. Better still, only a handful of people were stage-managing opera at the time, so she knew she "could always find work." And find work she did, as the above biography proves. In fact, her work in the theater has left little time to pursue other passions.

Linda has never married, although she still sees a man whom she once dated regularly. "I'm one of those people who was married to my work. At this point, I'm not sure that I was meant to live with someone. I am involved in a people business, and when I get home, I need to recharge after the intensity of the day's work. The job is exhausting and takes up what you would otherwise give to a partner ... Some of my need to nurture is fulfilled by opera summer camp. We have kids between eight and 11 years old, and it lasts four weeks. Some of the little boys ..." She threw back her head and laughed, before continuing. "They are not embarrassed to dance, so they are *right there* with the choreography. They crack me up."

When asked if she would choose her life again, she paused a few moments before answering, "Yeah, probably. Some of my choices might have been different. And I have some ... well, some curiosity about how things might have turned out."

In a later conversation, Linda said, "I love producing shows. I love being in the theater. I agree with a friend who says that the worst day on the stage is better than the best day in the office. For me, sitting in the house on opening night is ... I don't even know how to describe it. There's some level on which, metaphorically, I don't exhale until the first round of applause. Then I feel like I can breathe out. When it's done right, there's no feeling quite like it."

Linda talked with her seven friends about their breast experiences before her initial appointments with the medical oncologist and the surgeon. She ultimately chose to have a wide local excision and chemotherapy, rather than a mastectomy. At the time of the wide local excision, an axillary sentinel lymph node biopsy was also done, which was immediately followed by removal of seven additional axillary lymph nodes, all of which were negative for metastatic carcinoma. (Sentinel lymph nodes are discussed in Chapter 6 about Twin Cities.)

Even though her lymph nodes were negative, Linda's oncologist recommended that she have adjuvant chemotherapy, radiation treatment, and five years of tamoxifen. While receiving chemotherapy, Linda moved in with her mother, who is a retired schoolteacher. "My mom was very calming. We never sat and talked about my breast cancer, but she was always just there as a support person. She didn't seem anxious, but then again, if there's stress in my mom's life, you'd never know it. She loves being a mom and she was so calming. I was lucky."

Linda's hair was beginning to grow back after finishing chemotherapy when she had her first post-treatment mammogram. The mammogram of the previously biopsied breast was negative; however, suspicious calcifications were seen in the opposite (contralateral) breast, which proved to be ductal carcinoma *in situ* (DCIS) or noninvasive carcinoma. This meant that the malignant tumor cells were still contained inside the ducts and had not yet spread into the fibrous and fatty tissues that surround the breast ducts. With the second diagnosis of malignancy in as many years, she met with a plastic surgeon and decided to have bilateral mastectomies with a transverse rectus abdominis myocutaneous (TRAM) flap reconstruction.

TRAM flaps are currently the most common pedicle (attached) muscle flap procedures used for breast reconstruction. The plastic surgeon excises a piece of skin, fat, and muscle from the lower abdomen and tunnels it under the skin to the chest where it is sewn in place at the mastectomy site(s). The original vessels of the lower abdomen that fed the now-transplanted tissue remain attached to the transplant to keep it alive in its new location.

Even though the recovery time from a TRAM flap is considerably longer than for implants or expanders, Linda chose the former because she didn't like the idea of something artificial in her body. "Because a TRAM flap is a one-time deal, I decided to have bilateral mastectomies. I had a friend who had a unilateral TRAM reconstruction and subsequently had cancer in the opposite breast. She wasn't a candidate for another TRAM."

Linda's first year of participating in the New York 3-Day was in 2000. When she asked her friend, Cheryl, for a donation, Cheryl said, "I won't give you money, but I'll walk with you." This meant, of course, that Cheryl would not only have to raise money but also walk 60 miles. The two women trained by walking in New York City. Linda said to Cheryl, "Remember? We went to the top of the Guggenheim and back down; to the museums; down to midtown Manhattan; shopping. The Bronx Zoo was great. We went to the park [Central Park] once, but walking around in a circle in a park was too boring. There are certainly more interesting places to walk in New York City than a park."

When asked if she thought the 3-Day route was interesting, Linda quipped, "Yeah, but they ought to rename it 'The Terrorist Walk.'" She was alluding to our route through all five boroughs of New York City, across bridges from which we were forbidden to take photographs, and across New York Harbor on the Staten Island Ferry, in full view of the Statue of Liberty, which had reopened that week for the first time since 9/11.

On Day 1, Opening Ceremonies were at Belmont Park in Queens; Pit Stops were at Cunningham Park and Fajardo Playground; as mentioned, lunch was at Corona Park, where I met Linda and Cheryl. We three finished the day's route together by crossing the Triborough Bridge (over the East River Suspension Bridge part) to Randall's Island. Most of the route was pleasant and interesting, especially the part that passed by the remains of the 1964 World's Fair; however, at the risk of breaking the 3-Day cardinal rule of "No Whining," I must say that the Triborough Bridge was scary. In the midportion of the 2.1-mile bridge, concrete dividers were all that separated pedestrians from fiercely driven cars and trucks. Even worse, the bridge *vibrated*. Granted, my West Texas desert upbringing may have had a part in my apprehension about bridges— after all, the only things suspended over air in the desert are the parallel metal pipes over the pits of cattle guards—but even Linda and Cheryl (two nimble New Yorkers) weren't thrilled about walking across the Triborough Bridge.

To be fair to the 3-Day organizers, walkers had the option to ride a sweep vehicle across bridges. Even so, one particularly determined walker asked other walkers to surround her and lead her across. She locked arms and held hands with two women on either side of her; a third woman was ahead of her; a fourth behind. The little congregation crossed the bridge—protecting and being protected. The scene's tenderness brought tears to my eyes. I remembered again what Howard Sitron had said: "The 3-Day is how we want the world to be."

The next morning, as many of us were taking down our tents, "The Star-Spangled Banner" suddenly struck up over the speakers. Every one of us immediately dropped what we were doing, turned to watch the flag being raised, and started singing. Instead of tepid singing, we raised our voices, and in place of the usual let's-get-the-game-started cheer at the end, there was silence. We stood still for about 15 seconds, facing the flag. We then returned to the task at hand, more quiet than before. This was, indeed, how I wanted the world to be.

On Day 2, we crossed back over the Triborough Bridge into Queens and headed toward the Pulaski Bridge, which would take us into Brooklyn. For this part of the route, I walked (or, rather, tried to keep pace) with a woman whom I had met the day before. She talked fast and walked even faster—as if she were trying to stay ahead of her sadness. She frequently became tearful as she told me the story of her older sister's death from breast cancer at age 50. Several times during our conversation, she paused, looked at me, smiled sadly, and told me how much I reminded her of her older sister. I didn't know what to say to that, but it did make me think—perhaps for the first time—about how sad my three younger sisters would have been if I had not been fortunate enough to be diagnosed early.

———

At my insistence, she left me behind at Pit Stop 1, which was at Astoria Park. She rushed on alone and I resumed my slow, steady pace. A few miles later, the route wound through Queensbridge Park, by baseball diamonds full of children getting dirty, making noise, and trying to please the parents who were watching. I was walking slowly enough for a memory about my husband, Andy, to catch up. After all, it was August 7, 2004—the fifth anniversary of his death from metastatic rectal cancer at age 47.

Andy was a superb high school athlete in the little town in West Texas where he grew up. He was an all-district football player and he ran track, but his best sport was baseball. He was such a standout that he received 12 college baseball scholarship offers; however, by the end of high school, he was tired of competitive sports and declined all offers—a decision that he was to regret. He played on his college fraternity teams, though, and later, when he was a student at St. Mary's Law School, he played on an intramural softball team.

To be sure, there were many remarkable moments in my husband's life, but if there was a defining moment, it might have been at an intramural softball game during his last semester at law school. Andy's team of senior law students was vying for the championship against another team of senior law students. It appeared that these students had learned their lessons well: The competition between these two teams of future lawyers was ferocious.

In this final softball game of the final semester, it was the bottom of the last inning, with two outs. Andy's team was trailing by three points with the bases loaded. It was Andy's turn at bat. He stepped up to the plate and swung through his strike zone. The pitcher wound up and threw. Ball one. A tipped foul. Ball two. Ball three. A swing and a miss. The count was full—three balls, two strikes. The fans were stamping their feet and shrieking. This was, after all, *it*.

At that moment—a sparkling, slow-motioned moment—Andy turned around, made eye contact with me, and winked. On the next pitch, he hit a grand slam home run to win the game. That happened on a spring afternoon in 1979 but, every time that memory catches up to me, it was only yesterday.

Andy was a charismatic and successful trial attorney, and he was never afraid to swing for the bleachers. Best of all, he had a terrific sense of humor. Even near the end, he made people laugh. A few hours before he slipped into a coma because of bleeding in a brain metastasis, I brought him lunch on a tray. His besieged brain did not allow him to recognize that what I had brought was one of his favorite meals, and he refused to eat. Noticing the untouched food, our then 14-year-old son, Andrew, asked him why he hadn't eaten. My emaciated, brave husband said, with a grin, "I'm going on a hunger strike." This is one of the many, many funny stories that my son tells (and retells) about his father, sometimes laughing so hard that tears roll down his cheeks.

The route took us over the East River from Brooklyn into the Lower East side of Manhattan by way of the Williamsburg Bridge. This bridge's utilitarian architecture is criticized by people who knowingly comment on such things, but its no-frills flatfootedness was reassuring to me. Besides, the pedestrian walkway was at a different level than the cars and trucks. I wasn't one bit afraid.

Later, as we walked through Manhattan's financial district toward the ferry, 10 blocks of Water Street were closed to traffic for a Hoop-It-Up basketball tournament. Shouted conversations between 3-Day walkers joined the barked instructions among players, the blaring music, and the loudspeaker announcements. Orange balls, brightly colored jerseys, and flashy booths almost obscured the 3-Day black route signs with their white arrows. It was like the 3-Day had temporarily blended into a delirious street party. I wanted to throw confetti and dance.

A short time later, we crossed New York Harbor on the Staten Island Ferry. That was, unequivocally, the most emotional part of the New York 3-Day for me—more so, even, than Opening and Closing Ceremonies. I couldn't help crying as I looked across the harbor at the Statue of Liberty, resplendent in the bright sunlight.

An August 4, 2004, article in *USA Today* by Christina Jeng entitled, "Reopened Lady Liberty Welcomes Back Hundreds," had reported: "The Statue of Liberty opened to hundreds of visitors Tuesday for the first time since the September 11 attacks and in the face of warnings over new attacks. Tight security and concerns about terrorist strikes on financial centers in Manhattan, Newark, N.J. and Washington, D.C., didn't dampen sprits on Liberty Island."

As I gazed back at the receding Manhattan skyline, I was humbled and honored to be among New Yorkers who, despite their fears, continued to watch their children play baseball and bounce basketballs in the streets of Manhattan and ride ferries and visit statues and play music on loudspeakers and cheer and leap and high-five and laugh and walk—yes, that, too—in the indomitable and singular city that they called home.

On Day 3, we crossed the Bayonne Bridge, which was even more frightening to me than the Triborough had been. The Bayonne Bridge passes over Kill van Kull (which joins New York Harbor and Newark Bay) and links Staten Island to the Bayonne peninsula of New Jersey. The pedestrian walkway is cantilevered from the primary roadway. This means that we walked on a narrow strip of sidewalk, which was held aloft and separated from the main part of the span by beams that jutted out from the side of the bridge. True, we were separated from the traffic, but we were separated by *air*. The whole setup didn't feel all that substantial. And the water was way, way down below us and very big, at least by West Texas standards. (Big water remains vaguely unsettling to me, still.) The vantage point—with buildings visible in every direction—was paradoxically claustrophobic.

Fortunately, I was walking with a man from New Jersey named Michael McCallion, Jr., 36, who was built like a linebacker. He offered to let me hold onto his arm when I told him I was afraid. I didn't take him up on his offer, but I felt protected all the same, knowing that I could grab his arm if I began to panic. Michael was walking slowly because of swollen, painful knees, so I caught up with him along the route on Sunday morning. We walked together until the lunch stop and were often passed by other walkers, some saying hello to him by name.

Michael was my next-flap (as in tent-flap) neighbor. The tents were inches apart, so I couldn't help but hear his side of cell phone conversations. At Camp One, Friday night, it sounded like he was talking to his wife. Telling her about his knees hurting, he said, "They give me some stuff like, you know, Ben Gay, but it don't smell bad like Ben Gay. Know what I'm saying?" His wife was apparently sympathetic and concerned, and he said, "Don't you be worrying about nothing there. They got doctors all over the place." On Saturday night, I overheard conversations with his children, who I later learned were 3 and 1 years old. It was obvious, from my unavoidable eavesdropping of his words and tone, that he missed them a lot. He later told me that, "My wife looks Italian, but the kids are all me. My wife, with the kids, you wouldn't know she was their mother. Thank God for my kids. I told my wife I wanted another one, and she said, well ..." He chuckled and added, "I won't tell you exactly what she said, but the answer was ... well, it was no."

Michael was walking in memory of his mother-in-law, Lillian Gambucci, who died from breast cancer in February 2004. She was 76 years old and a widow when she was taken to the emergency room by her family for shortness of breath. One of her daughters was in the exam room with her mother and was shocked when the Emergency Room doctor pulled aside her mother's hospital gown, revealing a swollen, bruised-appearing breast. It was soon determined that she had locally advanced breast cancer with widely metastatic disease to the lungs, bones, and brain. Despite aggressive treatment, she died within months of presentation.

I asked Michael why he thought she waited so long before seeking treatment, and he said that she was probably embarrassed. He described his mother-in-law, whom he clearly loved and admired, as being proud and never wanting to be a burden to her children. She and her late husband were from Italy and, although she didn't drive, she went to work on an assembly line, setting screws to support their family, after her husband was disabled by a massive heart attack. Still, in many ways she was old-fashioned; she certainly didn't discuss her private body parts with anyone.

Her reticence sometimes complicated the family's attempts to discuss treatment options with the doctors and among themselves. "It was a very, very touchy situation. You couldn't really get too much into detail. You had to be careful what you said in front of her so's you wouldn't embarrass her." Also, Michael didn't get to visit her in the hospital nearly as much as he would have liked, which he now feels guilty about. "I know she didn't want to cry in front of us, and she didn't want us to see her in pain, you know? To see her like that hurt me a lot, and I didn't want her to feel uncomfortable. You knew she was in pain. You knew she didn't want to talk about it. You knew she just wanted to be left alone." Michael paused to compose himself. He cleared his throat before continuing, his voice husky. "You don't know what to do. There's nothing you can do. You don't want it to be happening. It got to the point where she had no hair, she had no breast, and she was so far gone that she needed to go home and pray to God that He would take her. Nobody deserves that."

When his mother-in-law was gravely ill, the medical oncologist came into the hospital room and reported that the cancer was progressing and that she needed more surgery. The nurse, who was standing at the bedside, whirled around and demanded, in front of Mrs. Gambucci and her family members, "What are you doing to this lady?" The doctor seemed surprised by the outburst. He looked first at the patient and then around the room at the family members before saying, "If the family agrees, I have no objection to giving her morphine and keeping her comfortable." She died two days later.

Michael said, "I believe they would have just kept doing operations. They were doing operation after operation after operation. Meanwhile, she was coming home and saying that it's in the lung, it's in the bone, it's in the brain. So why were they doing operations? It may have had some part in doing research or something. I really don't know. If you bring anything up to them, then they feel like you're telling them they're doing something wrong or they should be doing something more, which wasn't really the case."

Michael's wife was only 36, but he said he was already urging her to get her first mammogram, rather than waiting until she was 40, and to eat a healthy diet. About cancer's etiology, he said, "I'm a firm believer that it's in your diet. You got to stay away from the sweets, the carbohydrates, and all that kind of crap. We've been living in Jersey for so long, and they've been dumping in Jersey for so long, it's a wonder we don't all have cancer." He shrugged his shoulders and raised his hands chest-high with the palms up in the whudayagonnado way that I'd seen on TV.

"I grew up in Toms River, which is a cancer cluster. I work for Emmanuel Cancer Foundation. I deliver the toys to the kids. I give them money without telling them; I just stick money in their door—not that I have a lot of money, but I give them what I can. One of the kids—Joey Rogers—he's 16 years old. He's got cancer so bad, he had to get all new teeth. It's horrible. You go to their house. They live in this crappy apartment in the middle of New Brunswick ... These people that work for Emmanuel Cancer work so hard. I mean these are *good* people. The director called us up like two weeks ago, and she says, like, 'Listen. We have this whole family, the kid's got cancer. They got no mattress. They're all sleeping on the floor.' So we had to go out, get a truck, go pick up the mattress. We couldn't get the truck for three days, so they went to one of the radio stations, and they donated the truck. I tell you. You think you have problems? You see these kids with cancer. It's sickening. You feel so ..." Michael shook his head.

"Helpless?" I suggested.

"Oh, yeah. What do you do? I couldn't imagine. God forbid."

I suggested that some people walked in the 3-Day because it was a way to feel less helpless. He agreed, and said, "I had so many people that donated and gave to me. I had one company—Wite Rose Foods—that everybody gave me a dollar and they could wear jeans any day they wanted. I got 400 from them, and I got a big donation from Rubachem Systems. I did good. I raised like 28 hundred bucks. I really didn't try all that hard. Next year, if I did it, I would try a lot harder. How could you not give? I never have understood people who don't.

"I tell people all the time, I tell my kids: You have to help people. If people need your help, you help them. You may not be able to do a lot, but at least you tried. I wouldn't do this again by myself, though. You find out that when you walk with people, like you said, you talk, you keep your mind off stuff, and everybody keeps moving. I have some people I work with that want to do it, and we're thinking about maybe starting a team."

What a good man. Like, a real good man. You know what I'm saying?

———

A 3-Day team doesn't have to be a group. It can be just two people, like the mother and daughter team of Louise and Kerri Goodall. I met Kerri Goodall, Louise Goodall's 21-year-old daughter, in the shower line. She overheard a conversation about the book project and said, "My mom is a survivor." She added that, as a 50th birthday present for her mother, she had signed up the two of them for the walk. She also said that her mother had just passed the five-year survival mark. She seemed so, so pleased that her mother had reached that milestone.

On the afternoon of Day 3, I saw Kerri at a Pit Stop. She introduced me to her mother as "the lady that I told you about from the shower line." They posed for a photograph as if I were one of their old war buddies.

Akin to the conversations between airplane seat mates who were originally strangers, the conversations between women waiting in the shower line—actually, a semicircle of plastic chairs—sometimes veered sharply and dove headfirst into amazingly personal subjects. Maybe this had something to do with just walking 20 miles and being dirty and tired and having hat hair and wearing flip-flops. It didn't matter which woman in the semicircle had been the prettiest at her senior prom, or the most dazzling on her wedding day, or the best dressed at the office party, because she was just as grungy as the rest of us. This was somehow liberating. During that 15- or 20-minute wait to take a hot shower in a semi-trailer, we were grizzled comrades sitting around the campfire, sharing tales of triumph and tragedy—or, rather, unvarnished stories about our families, particularly our husbands and ex-husbands, and, in the case of the younger women, their parents, particularly their mothers.

In the holding area, while waiting for Closing Ceremonies to begin, I established a ritual that I was to follow at all the remaining 3-Day events, except Arizona: I took a nap.

At Liberty State Park in New Jersey, one of the white tents was designated as the gathering area for the survivors. Louise Goodall and Linda Jackson were there. So were about 60 other survivors. While we waited, I spread out my souvenir pink survivor's t-shirt on the grass and, using my fanny pack as a pillow and my cap as an eye shade, curled up and went to sleep. Despite booming music and exuberant conversations among the finishers, I slept soundly.

When I awoke, Barbara Jo and Bob Kirshbaum were a few feet away, sitting vigil. Bob said that I had been lying so still that he had become concerned about me. (He may have been kidding. Sometimes I couldn't tell if Bob was kidding.) Even so, it was comforting that these two kind people had been watching over me.

Barbara Jo and Bob are from Upland, California. Barbara Jo is a legendary long-distance walker for breast cancer. She participated in her first 3-Day event in 1998 and, by the end of the 2004 Komen 3-Day and Avon 2-Day seasons, had completed 42 long-distance walking events and raised nearly half a million dollars for the breast cancer cause. Remarkably, none of the money she raised was from corporations. While Barbara Jo walked in events, Bob's self-assigned job was to post bright pink "Team California" signs along the entire route. The signs had encouraging and often humorous messages. Barbara Jo sometimes gently touched Bob's signs as she passed by, smiling to herself.

Prior to the first 2004 3-Day event in Boston, Barbara Jo had called me when she noticed my name on the group e-mailings for participants in multiple 3-Day events. When we met, Barbara Jo, Bob, and I became fast friends. Over the next three months— August, September, and October 2004—I grew to love them like they were family. (Barbara Jo even indulged my request to let me call her "my big sister." Carrying that guise further, we pretended that Bob and Barbara Jo's daughter, Debra, was named after me.) Playfulness aside, it is not an overstatement that I could not, *could not*, have completed all 10 events or written this book without their support and encouragement and senses of humor.

Also, the fact that Bob (Robert J. Kirshbaum, M.D.) is an internist comforted my mother immeasurably. The four episodes of pneumonitis (lung inflammation) that I mentioned in Chapter 1 caused irreversible lung scarring. Since then, I have carefully avoided situations that might trigger another episode. (After all, I don't want to end up wheeling around an oxygen tank with tubes up my nose.) Before the walks even started, I had to contend with my mother's concern about my sleeping in a tent during cold or rainy weather. She was afraid I would get gravely ill and—to continue the melodramatic tone—be all alone in a strange city. With Bob and Barbara Jo Kirshbaum along, I was far, far from alone. She may have been immeasurably relieved but, truth told, so was I.

When bad weather forced me to forgo camping and stay in a hotel, Bob made reservations for me at the same place that he and Barbara Jo were staying and gave me a ride back and forth. Barbara Jo camped at 3-Day events in previous years, but about sleeping in tents again in 2004, she said, "Been there, done that." During the 2004 3-Day events, she and Bob always stayed in hotels, and I had a standing invitation to come along, whether or not it was cold or rainy.

It also became a standing date for Barbara Jo and me to meet at lunchtime on the third day of each event and walk the last leg together. Even when some of their grown children joined them for the walks, I was still included in all the Kirshbaum family activities. They even convinced me to help carry the "Team California" banner as we finished 3-Day events together across the country. (You must understand that to carry a banner with another state's name is a monumental concession for a Texan. *Monumental.*)

After Closing Ceremonies, I overheard the single funniest conversation of the New York 3-Day when I was on the shuttle bus headed toward the hotel. A woman with a pronounced New York accent said, "I've been nice to everyone for three days. Please, this. Thank you, that. Did you see the looks we were getting in the Bronx when we were saying, 'Good morning'? I've never in my life said '*Good morning*' to someone in the Bronx. Being this nice is not *normal*. I don't know about you, but I can't wait to get back to the city so I can be pissy again."

The woman beside her said, "I hear what you're saying."

Despite my wobbly imitation of a New York accent, when I repeated that conversation to the folks back home, it never failed to evoke belly laughs and knee slaps. After all, the anecdote supported the Texas notion that the border river that needs guarding is not the Rio Grande but the Red (the one along the northeastern border of the state).

Relax, everyone. That's a *joke*. Hear what I'm saying?

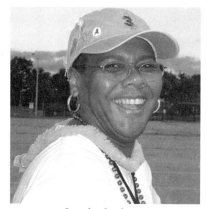

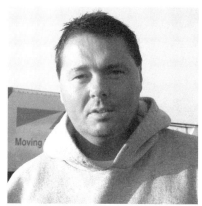

Linda Jackson   *Michael McCallion, Jr.*

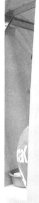

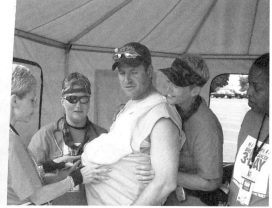

Medical crew

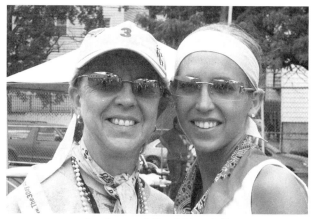

Louise and Kerri Goodall

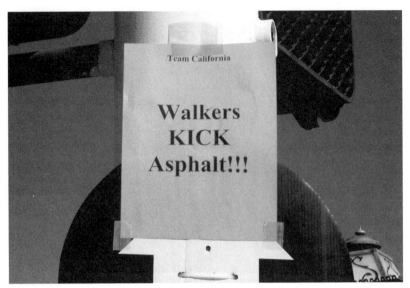

A Team California sign

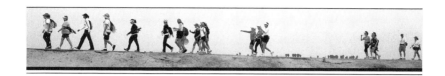

Chapter 3

Washington, D.C.

August 13, August 14, and August 15, 2004

An Internet article about the upcoming annual Perseid meteor shower on August 12, 2004, assured us that "new data and calculations" repudiate the 1992 prediction that Comet Swift-Tuttle (the source of the meteor shower) will collide with Earth in the year 2126 and result in a die-off of dinosaur-sized proportions. In the June 25, 2004 article, Bill Cooke of the National Aeronautics and Space Administration (NASA) Marshall Space Flight Center explained why 2004 was going to be a good year for Perseids. "First, the Moon is new in mid-August; moonlight won't spoil the show. Second, in addition to the usual shower on August 12, there *might be* an extra surge of meteors on August 11, caused by a filament of dust newly drifting across Earth's orbit … *If predictions are correct,* Earth will plow through the filament on Wednesday, August 11, at 2100 UT (5 PM EDT)." [Emphasis added.]

The italics are mine, as is this question: If the rocket scientists at NASA are waffling about an extra surge of meteors six *weeks* hence, how can they be cocksure about Comet Swift-Tuttle's whereabouts 122 *years* from now? And, while I'm knocking governmental agencies, why didn't the National Weather Service meteorologists do better at predicting Hurricane Charley's path in August 2004? Or, for that matter, why wasn't there so much as a peep from them about the hail storm slated for the afternoon of August 11, 2004, in Chantilly, Virginia, a suburb of Washington, D.C.? A hail storm that would—if my childhood memories serve me correctly—rival those in West Texas.

The explanation, of course, is that a comet's dust trail and a hurricane's path and the collision of updrafts and downdrafts that will spew hail stones are capricious. Scientists merely base their predictions on collected data that are extrapolated from sophisticated and complex calculations—in other words, they make educated guesses. Time and chance are, after all, happening. The same is true when speculating about an individual's chance of surviving breast cancer.

When Carolynn Johnson, 41, was diagnosed with breast cancer in November 2000, an oncologist in another state to whom she was sent for a second opinion gave her an educated forecast. The news was not only frightening but, to Carolynn's ear, brutally conveyed. "Almost the first thing she [the oncologist] said was, 'I want you to know that your chances of being alive in five years are only 60%.' Then she pulls out this big paper and proceeds to tell me that there's a such-and-such chance that the chemo will make me sterile. I'm sitting there thinking, We're going to get through this one day at a time. We're *going* to get through this. Even if she felt the need to give me statistics, she could have concentrated on how many people survive rather than die."

Carolynn had Stage II disease, meaning that her tumor was less than 5 cm in greatest dimension and her axillary lymph nodes were negative for metastatic carcinoma. Patients with Stage II disease are generally considered to have an excellent chance of long-term survival. So why did the consulting medical oncologist tell her that her chance of survival for five years was only 60%? Well, because Carolynn had a complicating medical condition. At the time she was diagnosed, she was pregnant.

In 2000, Carolynn was 37 years old and living a peaceful life in North Tazewell, Virginia, with her husband, Frank, and their two-year-old daughter, Abigail. One evening while she was lying in bed, their little dog jumped on the bed and bumped her chest, causing a sharp pain. When she rubbed the spot, she was surprised to find a lump beneath the skin. "At the time, I didn't know that I was pregnant, and I thought it was just a knot or a cyst. I was not at all alarmed. When a home pregnancy test indicated that I was pregnant, I made a mental note to have the OB check my breast when I went in for the first appointment. Because of my age and the media saying that mammograms are unnecessary until age 40, I never gave any thought to the possibility of the lump being cancer. Still, I knew that the lump shouldn't be ignored, so I called my doctor's attention to it when I went in. In the two and a half weeks between the first time I felt it and when I went to see the OB, the lump had tripled in size. When the doctor felt the lump, though, he said it didn't feel like anything to be alarmed about. To be sure, he sent me for an ultrasound that very day and referred me to a surgeon.

"I returned to the surgeon's office four days later for the results, and the surgeon said, 'We're going to do a biopsy.' The biopsy was scheduled for two days later. I left the surgeon's office and went straight to the hospital and preregistered for surgery. Throughout this time I remained calm. At no point did I even consider the possibility that the lump was cancer. I have a strong faith in God and reasoned that He had given me the gift of a surprise, unplanned pregnancy. Surely, I reasoned, this lump wouldn't be cancer. God wouldn't let it be cancer. Besides, if I hadn't been pregnant, my breasts wouldn't have been tender, and I wouldn't have felt the mass and sought evaluation ... I believe God gifted me with pregnancy, giving me tender breasts. If it weren't for being pregnant, I might not have felt the lump. I might have waited until it was too late."

Carolynn's father is the pastor of Calvary Baptist Chapel, so her faith in God might be thought of as a birthright. Furthermore, she is both literally and figuratively close to her father, since she lives next door to her parents. About her father, she says, "I'm the oldest child and the only daughter. We're very close. He says, 'Other than my relationship with my wife, no one is closer to me than my daughter.' I hug him just like I was 12 years old." Even so, the story behind Carolynn's love for God and for her parents and, for that matter, for her husband, was not as open-textured as one might assume. The surface clues were her burgundy-dyed hair, bright blue fingernails, and an ankle tattoo.

Carolynn was 10 years old when her father began attending church. Prior to that, he did not go to church with the rest of the family; however, Carolynn later learned that he stood outside his children's doors and listened to their prayers at night. "We said, 'God, help Daddy to go to church with us,' because Mom taught us to do that. We didn't know until much later that it was making an impact on him. He ended up going to church and getting more and more involved, then became involved in the youth ministry and became an associate pastor. When he first started church work, he kept his job [in the mining industry] and didn't take a salary from the church until he could build up his ministry. While he was pastoring, he got his doctorate. Our family did not know that he was working on it, so it was a surprise when he showed us the certificate. We were all so proud of him." Carolynn smiled broadly, revealing beautiful teeth, her brown eyes sparkling.

When asked if she was a typical "preacher's kid," Carolynn looked away, her broad smile replaced by a pensive one. She paused, before continuing, as if choosing her words carefully. "I probably lived my late 20s like a lot of people live their teen-age years. There's no other way to say that. When I was home and Dad was involved with the ministry, there were a lot of things that I was not permitted to do. In hindsight, it did not hurt me in any way that I wasn't allowed to do certain things. Dad did what he believed was the right thing to do at the time. As he was learning his way, I didn't experience much as a teen-ager. I certainly don't have any regrets.

"When I met Frank [her husband], I knew it was the way love was supposed to feel. I was 32 and had been living on my own. All my friends knew me as a strong, independent, almost hard person. When I met Frank, everything changed." She flashed another smile. "Something about him softened me and made me another person ... I had gotten out of the church for a few years, and I recommitted myself and went home, and it was all good again." Carolynn nodded her head slowly and pressed her lips, like she might begin to cry.

"Living several states away, there was a period of time that I didn't even come home to visit. I had left the church and wasn't living as I should have been. He [her father] didn't preach to me as far as 'You should do this' or 'You should do that.' That was not my dad. I just stayed away because I was living a different life, and I wouldn't shame him. I would not do anything to harm his ministry. I called three or four times a year. When I called and told them that I had met someone, he said, 'What is past is past, Carolynn.' He knew, and believed, that I was making a positive change in my life. Frank and I started visiting my parents once a month, and it got to the point that when we'd leave, I would start to cry driving down the road, because it was so comfortable there ... About a year after Frank and I got together, we quit our jobs [in Charlotte] and moved back. We've been there seven years now. It's a good life."

When I mentioned the similarity between her homecoming story and the New Testament parable about the prodigal son, Carolynn began to nod before I even finished the sentence, as if she had considered it often. "The story of the ultimate father's love applies. When I hear that story—when Dad brings that story into the sermon—what is central to the story has nothing to do with the child leaving home, but that the father gave him his half and let him go, and after all the bad stuff that the son had done, the father waited at the fence for him to come home and then put a robe on him."

Actually, the future husband who helped Carolynn "come to herself" (to borrow an idiom from the Scripture about the prodigal son) was a longtime acquaintance. She had met Frank through his older brother, Drew, when Frank was 18 and she was 25. About their reintroduction, seven years later, she said, "He was grown up, and he wasn't a kid anymore. It was instant. There was a moment when we were talking that our eyes locked, and I was gone." Carolynn rolled her eyes, shook her head, and laughed. "That was it. I was later told that, after I left his shop, Frank went out to some of his employees and said, 'I'm going to marry that girl,' and he did. We were married within six months. It was absolutely, without a doubt, right."

Carolynn and Frank's first daughter was born two years after they were married. They thought their family was complete, so the second pregnancy was a surprise, just days after Carolynn discovered the breast mass. She was seven weeks pregnant at the time of the breast biopsy and opted for local anesthesia because of concern about the effect of general anesthesia on the developing fetus. This meant, of course, that she was awake during the biopsy procedure. The surgeon had previously told her that he was planning to do a frozen section on the tissue, and the only conversation that she remembered from the procedure concerned the biopsy tissue being sent to Pathology. As mentioned in the last chapter, a frozen section on the tissue allowed the surgeon to know the results almost immediately.

Since she didn't have general anesthesia, Carolynn went directly to her hospital room after the procedure without first going to the Recovery Room. She waited so long for her husband and father to come to her room that she began to worry that the two men had mistakenly thought she was going to the Recovery Room. After what seemed to her an inordinate wait, her father, her husband, and the surgeon arrived. She laughed and said, "I thought you guys had forgotten about me."

Her father replied, "No, we didn't forget about you."

As the men gathered at her bedside, they seemed to be acting normal. In retrospect, Carolynn realized that they were trying to hide their feelings. The surgeon was the first to speak. "I'm afraid the news is not so good, Carolynn. It's cancer."

Carolynn looked at her father, who was standing at the foot of her bed, and saw tears coming to his eyes. She then looked at her husband, who was beside her. He had begun to cry as well. The surgeon spoke again: "We recommend that you have an abortion." He then told her that an oncologist would be coming by to visit her later.

Carolynn remembered shaking her head and saying, "It's too much. I can't make the decision. I need to let it sink in." She realized that her legs were trembling.

Later that day, Dr. Mario Stefanini, an 81-year-old medical oncologist from Richlands, Virginia, visited Carolynn. "As soon as he walked in the room, I had a feeling of peace and immediate trust. Dr. Stefanini had already been online and had called [M.D.] Anderson. He told me that the abortion decision could be postponed until the final pathology was out. People later asked me if I was going to Winston-Salem [the nearest referral oncology center]. They would ask me, 'Are you going here? Are you going there?' I had a local doctor who, before he ever laid eyes on me, had gone online to look at the research about pregnancy and breast cancer."

Dr. Stefanini might have called M.D. Anderson Cancer Center in Houston because of the retrospective study of pregnant women diagnosed with breast cancer, which was underway at that institution. Between 1986 and 2001, 39 pregnant women were diagnosed with breast cancer and treated at Anderson. Dr. L.P. Middleton and her coauthors subsequently reported their results in the medical journal *Cancer* in 2003. Their evaluation confirmed previous studies that showed pregnancy's negative effect on overall survival. Only 22 (56%) of the women were alive with no evidence of disease during a mean follow-up period of 43 months.

The day following surgery, Carolynn, her husband, and her father met with the surgeon and Dr. Stefanini to discuss the pathology results.

"We were told that the cancer was very aggressive; invasive; the nerves were unrecognizable. It was unsure whether the margins were negative. They recommended a modified radical mastectomy. I never hesitated. I was also told that the status of the lymph nodes would determine whether the pregnancy would be allowed to continue."

The meeting with the medical oncologist was on a Friday, and the surgery was scheduled for the following Monday. Over the weekend, Carolynn and her family tried to "operate normally." Most of the congregation at Calvary Baptist Chapel had already learned about Carolynn's diagnosis through the prayer line, but her father announced from the pulpit that Carolynn had cancer and asked everyone to pray that the axillary lymph nodes would be free of cancer.

In less than two weeks, Carolynn went from being a joyful obstetrical patient to having a mastectomy and becoming a cancer patient. "Everything happened so fast. I was told that during the mastectomy an abortion could occur as a result of the anesthesia. I had difficulty with the idea that I might be faced with the decision of whether or not to terminate the pregnancy. The idea that I might lose my baby was much more acceptable than having an abortion—*to have to make that choice.*"

———

The general anesthesia that was required for the mastectomy and lymph node dissection did not cause a miscarriage, and Carolynn was discharged from the hospital a day after surgery. She spent the next two days at her parents' house. "I had two drains and was wrapped in an Ace® bandage. In the hospital, I could look down, and it wasn't obvious that part of me was missing. Before surgery, I was barely a 'C' cup. I asked Mom to change the bandage. I was afraid to look under the bandage. I was concerned about it being bloody or gory. I wasn't worried that a part of me was missing."

Carolynn's husband Frank emptied the drains and her mother changed the bandage. "When she [Carolynn's mother] took off the bandage the first time, she said, 'This is really not bad.' When I looked down, I was shocked at what I saw. There was a long incision, real clean, with only one drop of blood. It was so clean that it wasn't scary ... It would have been helpful for someone to explain to me what to expect when the bandage was changed."

Her axillary lymph nodes were negative for metastatic carcinoma, so she was spared the decision about undergoing a therapeutic abortion in order to immediately begin chemotherapy. (It turned out that lymphatic invasion was present in the breast tissue.) Instead, she was able to postpone chemotherapy until after the first trimester of her pregnancy. She then received four cycles of Adriamycin® and Cytoxan® at three-week intervals. Like nearly every cancer patient who receives this combination, she lost most of her hair after the first cycle. As a show of solidarity, her husband, her father, and her younger brothers shaved their heads. Her father, who had started growing a beard, even shaved that off.

Although Carolynn's mother didn't symbolically shave her head, she helped in a more concrete way by taking care of Carolynn and Frank's two-year-old daughter during the day. Frank also shouldered most of the household responsibilities. "Chemo took me down. It just took me down. I was on the couch a lot of the time. Frank would get up, go to work, come home, stand in the kitchen and eat something, take care of Abigail, clean the house, do the laundry, give me a rub, put me to bed, keep on cleaning, get up, and do it again. My parents were great about taking care of Abigail. My husband and my parents made it possible for me to only do one thing, and that was to recover … My only responsibility was to get through chemotherapy and to get well."

Hannah Elizabeth Stephanie (in honor of Dr. Stefanini) Johnson was born on July 24, 2001. Four weeks after she delivered a healthy baby girl, Carolynn received the first of what was initially scheduled to be four additional courses of combination chemotherapy (epirubicin, fluorouracil, cyclophosphamide, and methotrexate). After the fourth postdelivery course of chemotherapy, her scans were clear, but her serum carcinoembryonic antigen (CEA) level remained slightly elevated. "Dr. Stefanini told me that we had come too far, and that we had to do everything we could to fight the cancer, so I had a fifth round."

CEA is a serum tumor marker that is useful for following some breast cancer patients. Before surgery, the elevation of CEA is stage-dependent. This means that serum CEA levels are elevated in 10% of women with Stage I breast cancer, 19% with Stage II, 31% with Stage III, and 64% with Stage IV. Five percent of women with benign breast lesions have elevated levels, too, but only about half of patients with recurrent breast cancer will have an increased CEA level. In other words, by itself, this lab test is not particularly reliable for either *detecting the presence* or *confirming the absence* of breast cancer; however, if an individual patient's serum level was increased before surgery, following the CEA level is one way to gauge her response to chemotherapy.

Another serum tumor marker that is useful in (again) some breast cancer patients is CA 15-3 antigen. It is elevated in about 30% of patients with known breast cancer and, like CEA, correlates with stage. Unfortunately, it is not a good screening test because only about 20% of patients with Stage I, II, and III disease have increased levels, and some patients without breast cancer have slightly elevated levels. CA 15-3 is better, though, than CEA at detecting recurrent disease, especially metastatic disease. Still, its best use, like that of CEA, is for gauging *response to treatment*. An increase in the CA 15-3 level by more than 25% in a patient with metastatic disease signals disease progression, while a decrease by more than 25% means that the patient's metastatic disease is responding to treatment. CA 27-29 is still another tumor marker, which is similar to CA 15-3. It is increased in about 40% of patients with known Stage I, II, and III disease.

Unfortunately, for both routine screening and surveillance of breast cancer patients, serum tumor markers are pretty crappy. (Sorry. I searched the thesaurus but couldn't find a word more precise than "crappy.") Studies have shown that patients without symptoms who have been followed with serum tumor markers have no survival advantage over those who haven't been followed with serum tumor markers but who develop symptoms. In other words, a positive test result only alerts the patient that something bad is going on; it doesn't improve the patient's chance of surviving that bad thing. (Now, that's *really* crappy.)

After the fifth round, Carolynn's CEA level was normal. She was ultimately glad that she was treated so aggressively. "I hear so many stories about people who haven't been treated aggressively. I would pay that year again in a minute. I felt like Dr. Stefanini took a personal interest in me. He was more than just my oncologist. I felt like he really did have a personal stake in my well-being."

Throughout her cancer experience, her family's support was constant and nearby, but there were many others who followed her Web page. Carolynn learned about the 3-Day through a magazine ad and, in November 2001 (a year after diagnosis), she signed up for the May 2002 Washington, D.C., event. She soon started an online journal—"Pink Ribbon Miracle" (www.pinkribbonmiracle.com)—to chronicle her breast cancer experience and her training for the 3-Day. "Carolynn's crew" soon emerged as a successful fundraising vehicle, due largely to Carolynn's online journal and the accompanying Web site. (In 2004, Carolynn's crew raised over $60,000.)

In May 2002—just five months after finishing chemotherapy— Carolynn, her brother, Michael, and her best friend, Kelle, participated in the Washington, D.C., 3-Day. One of the high points for Carolynn was sharing her story on stage. She said that she was able to tell her story without crying, but she saw many in the audience moved to tears. She intended to participate the following year, in 2003; however, it was not to be.

Backing up a little: After Carolynn finished her final round of chemotherapy, she began taking tamoxifen. After several months, she developed abnormal uterine bleeding, which is a common side effect of tamoxifen treatment. Although tamoxifen-associated bleeding is usually due to benign causes, it can be due to cancer of the endometrium (the lining of the uterus). To rule this out, Carolynn had a diagnostic endometrial biopsy. The tissue was benign but, before long, she had a second bout of abnormal vaginal bleeding, which necessitated another biopsy. It too was benign but, to obviate repeated endometrial biopsies, Carolynn's gynecologist recommended a hysterectomy and bilateral salpingoophorectomy (removal of the uterus with the attached ovaries and fallopian tubes).

This major surgical procedure was added to the growing list of body blows that had begun with a breast biopsy, followed by a modified radical mastectomy and axillary node removal, four rounds of combination chemotherapy during her pregnancy, the delivery of a term baby, five more rounds of combination chemotherapy, tamoxifen treatment, and two diagnostic endometrial biopsies. Oh, yes. Between the last round of chemotherapy and the first endometrial biopsy, she trained for and participated in her first 60-mile walk. After the hysterectomy, Carolynn started a low carbohydrate diet and began training for her second 3-Day, which finally tipped the balance.

"I would all of a sudden feel like my heart was racing or fluttering and get light-headed and feel so fatigued. I kept thinking, Chemo was so long ago, so why is it that I'm worse than ever before? I did not accept the toll on my body of pregnancy, chemo, delivery, hysterectomy ... The fatigue got to the point where I couldn't leave the house for more than an hour ... Then there was the mental battle: Am I totally losing it here? Am I going to turn into an invalid? Am I going to be unable to leave my house? It scared me that I was becoming so insecure. I couldn't understand why it was happening at that stage. Why now?"

She talked to Dr. Stefanini about her symptoms. He, of course, ordered tests to rule out recurrent cancer. When those tests were negative, he pointed out how much her body had been through over the past few years. He offered antidepressant medication (which she declined) and urged her to rest. "I immediately went home and took two weeks off and just allowed my body to rest ... At the end of this time, I did start feeling better. I was still concerned about whether I would be able to travel to the [2003] 3-Day. Frank is my security blanket. The thought of having to leave home and not have him with me made me even more afraid. He stepped up to the plate and said, 'I'll go. We'll work it out. I'll go.'"

Frank and Carolynn attended the 2003 Washington, D.C., 3-Day and cheered for Carolynn's teammates—that is, as much as her health allowed her. Carolynn's health slowly improved over the following months, and her energy and enthusiasm returned. She vowed to walk in the next Washington, D.C., 3-Day, which was scheduled for August 2004. Her training was going well until May 2004, when a 1.5-cm mass was discovered in the contralateral (opposite) breast during a routine follow-up mammogram. (Although Carolynn didn't use this particular expression, I often heard women refer to the opposite, remaining breast as "the good side" and the side where the cancer was found as "the bad side.")

The mass had not been seen on imaging studies the previous September. In "Pink Ribbon Miracle," she wrote, "The final ultrasound report came back, and there are indicators that the cancer may have returned. I am a 4 on a scale of 5, with 5 being most probably malignancy. The undefined margins of this growth are also suspicious."

Even before the contralateral mass was discovered, Carolynn had been debating a prophylactic mastectomy of her remaining breast. She described the "urge" to pursue the mastectomy as a "whisper from God." She had already discussed the indications with her surgeon and her oncologist, and had made overtures to the insurance company for coverage of the elective procedure. With the new finding on her mammogram, her decision became clear-cut. "Do a mastectomy. Do it now."

In mid-June 2004, less than two months before the Washington, D.C., 3-Day, Carolynn underwent a simple mastectomy, which involved removal of nipple and areola, with an ellipse of surrounding skin, and underlying breast tissue. The axillary lymph nodes were not removed—the distinction from a modified radical mastectomy.

Carolynn and I laughed about the phrase "simple mastectomy." We took no umbrage from terms like "radical mastectomy" and "modified radical mastectomy" or the various terms for breast conservation treatment: "lumpectomy," "wide local excision," and "partial mastectomy." But "*simple*"? We wanted to know whom, exactly, it was simple for? Just because Carolynn was gritty enough to walk in the 3-Day less than two months after a *simple* mastectomy did not mean it was a trivial procedure. (We voted that the procedure's name be changed to "total mastectomy.")

The surgeon sent the simple/total mastectomy specimen for a frozen section and, as had been the case with the first breast biopsy, Carolynn learned the results shortly after the procedure was completed. When she learned the results this second time, she was still groggy from general anesthesia. In "Pink Ribbon Miracle," she wrote, "My brain was alert, and I could hear everything that was being said around me. With the anesthesia still in my system, I couldn't, however, make myself utter a word. I remember my grandmother telling me she loved me, and I could hear her crying. My dad leaned close and asked if I had spoken to the doctor. I slowly shook my head no. 'Do you want to know the results?' With a struggle, I slowly mumbled, 'All clear.' My dad smiled and said, 'Benign, Carolynn, all clear.' I struggled to speak again. 'Thank the Lord.'"

A "Pink Ribbon Miracle" post a week after her second mastectomy demonstrated, once again, the willingness of breast cancer patients to tell their stories as a way to help others. In fact, Carolynn went a brave step further:

Throughout the journey I have taken with this illness, I have encountered so many people, men and women alike, who envision a mastectomy as surgery that mutilates the body. I have given a lot of thought about this and have made a decision to "come out," so to speak, with my body. In doing so, I hope I will calm the fears that many people have. For those who have seen the scars, the response is one of surprise. It isn't "as bad" as they thought. I am most certain that the image the mind

creates is often worse than reality. For me, reconstruction was never a consider-
ation. A disease left me scarred. Those scars are here, but I am alive. I accept my
body as it is. After two mastectomies and a hysterectomy, I am no less a woman
than I was before my illness. I also have to say that I totally support a woman's right
to have breast reconstruction. Every individual has a different life situation, and
different views or perceptions of what is best for their own body ...

At the end of the post, she invited readers to see for themselves. "These pictures were taken last night, six days post-op: *click here to view*; close up: *click here to view.*"

Carolynn's unblinking acceptance of scars (or "wounds," as she sometimes called her surgical incisions) was informed by more than her own experience with scars from her two mastectomies and hysterectomy. In fact, her husband's disfigurement from a childhood accident may have been the "different life situation" to which she was alluding. Excerpting her post and taking the liberty of adding italics and changing pronouns gives still deeper insight into Carolynn's coping style: "A *disease* left *him* scarred. Those scars are here, but *he is* alive. *He* accepts *his* body as it is." Put another way, Carolynn had a mentor for accepting her body.

When Frank was four years old, he strayed too close to a kerosene-fueled brush fire and was badly burned on his face. The burns were so extensive that his eyesight, sense of smell, and ability to hear were thought to be in jeopardy; however, he recovered from the burns with all his senses intact, despite his face being disfigured. As he grew into a man, he was unapologetic about his severely scarred face. Carolynn said, "That was one of the things that impressed me about him most. He would walk into a place, head held high, speak to strangers. The scars have never been an issue for him. Those scars don't define him. They're not who he is. Just like I didn't deserve breast cancer, he didn't deserve to be burned as a child."

After her simple/total mastectomy, Carolynn resumed training for the 3-Day despite a drain that remained sutured in place for 10 days after surgery, an Ace® wrap that retarded fluid accumulation (but also restricted deep breathing), hot flashes, gastric reflux problems, and the double whammy of heat and humidity (a weather combination that she called her "nemesis"). Despite these obstacles, she persisted. To avoid the summer heat, she walked early in the day, whenever possible. Otherwise, she used a treadmill and, within a month after surgery, she was again able to walk 10 miles at a stretch. As the 3-Day approached, she felt increasingly confident that she would be able to join her D.C. teammates ... And join them she did.

For the event, Carolynn decided to pace herself so that she could walk a portion of the route on each of the three days. On Friday (Day 1), she walked 15 miles; on Saturday (Day 2), 11 miles; and, on Sunday (Day 3), 13 miles. On Days 1 and 3, the heat was the limiting factor; on Day 2, it was the rain.

Like the New York 3-Day being dubbed "The Terrorist Walk" because of the aforementioned Orange Alert, the Washington, D.C., 3-Day was nicknamed "The Hurricane Walk" because of the threat of rain and wind. The day before the walk began, Hurricane Charley's predicted path was less than a hundred miles west of our starting point at Dulles Expo Center in Chantilly, Virginia, and the planned route through the northern Virginia neighborhoods. Charley was expected to bring up to 7 inches of rain and wind gusts up to 50 mph. We were lucky, though. By the time the Category 4 hurricane reached the D.C. area, it had tilted east and deflated. It was little more than a summer shower by Saturday afternoon when it grazed the 3-Day route along Lake Accotink in North Springfield, Virginia. We didn't know that, though, when we started Day 2.

The morning of Day 2, an orange-shirted motorcycle safety crew volunteer told us about the day's route as we waited for the light to turn at a major street crossing: "You're going to turn right here and go up to Merrifield, across the Beltway. We'll walk a little through Falls Church, Greenway Downs; cross 50 into Annandale. Annandale Road lines a little neighborhood. Across 236; right on Americana; footbridge over into Wakefield Park; cross Braddock—not walk on it. Mile-and-a-half walk through Lake Accotink that will finish in the neighborhood of Irving Middle School." When the light changed, and we started to cross, someone asked the volunteer about the weather forecast. She grinned and said, "That's not my department."

That afternoon, I was glad for the three pounds of rain gear that I had been lugging around all day. Otherwise, it's likely that I would have joined those who had sense enough to come in out of the rain and boarded a camp-bound bus at the Ravensworth Elementary School Pit Stop at mile 15. Instead, I sloshed on and arrived at Irving Middle School in Fairfax, Virginia—the end of the day's route—remarkably dry. Instead of pitching tents in the mud, the 3-Day organizers opted to bus participants back to the Dulles Expo Center for what was billed as "the world's largest indoor slumber party." The following morning, walkers were bused back to Irving Middle School to resume the walk.

Day 2 of the Washington, D.C., walk was one of the few times during the 2004 3-Day season that I actually needed full rain gear. (The other times were in Chicago and San Francisco.) I packed the rain gear—a two-piece rain suit and galoshes—only when a soaking rain was likely because of its extra weight in my larger-than-usual fanny pack.

During the 600 miles of 2004 3-Days, I was asked, literally, hundreds of times what I was carrying in my fanny pack. I always carried a water bottle; a protein bar; a lightweight rain poncho; an extra pair of socks; sunscreen; lip balm; lip antioxidant (a gift from my gynecologist); Visine®; and a zippered, 8x10-inch, seven-ring Day-Timer®, which contained July, August, September, and October month-in-view calendar pages (filled with airline and hotel reservation information), address pages (to record contact information), plastic pouches and sleeves for my driver's license, credit card, health insurance card, medical license, extra business cards, money, photos of Tom and my children and my dogs, Brush-Ups® ("Clean Teeth, Fresh Breath, Anytime, Anywhere! Textured Teeth Wipes"), shuttle passes, a house key (for the Monday afternoons that I took a cab from the San Antonio International Airport back to my deliciously quiet, cool, blinds-drawn-for-a-nap, empty house), and extra memory chips. The Day-Timer®'s Velcro™-fastened side pocket contained (and protected) a digital camera; a voice recorder; a lapel microphone; my cell phone; two fresh AA batteries; roller ball pens; and a tiny Ziploc® bag with my lunchtime dose of vitamins, chelated minerals, and glucosamine chondroitin sulfate.

On Sunday afternoon, Carolynn's husband and daughters drove to D.C. from North Tazewell and met her at the Cora Kelly School Pit Stop in Alexandria, Virginia. She rode with them to the Closing Ceremonies holding area at the District of Columbia Superior Courthouse. She and her family joined the cheering crowd who was welcoming the 1,100 walkers as they arrived at the holding area. Among the walkers were Carolynn's 3-Day teammates. After the announcement directing families and friends to leave the holding area and go to the stage area, Carolynn parted with Frank and her daughters and joined the other "pinkies," as the survivors were called, to wait for the march down Pennsylvania Avenue.

I roused from my now-customary after-walk nap about the time the others were lining up three by three. I hurried—relatively speaking, since I was stiff and sore—to the pinkie gathering area near the base of the J.J. Darlington Memorial Statue—a gold-leafed representation of the nude goddess Diana standing beside a fawn. Someone had playfully dressed the statue in a pink survivor's t-shirt. I drowsily scanned the gathering of about 50 pink-shirted women for Carolynn but didn't see her.

It was then that I saw Monica Cooper, standing a few inches taller than most of the other women, also scanning the crowd. I had met Monica and her husband, Dale, on Day 2, and they had shared their story while we walked. When she spotted me, her eyes crinkled and she waved. I waved back. She worked her way through the close-shouldered crowd, hugged me, and asked, almost shyly, "Will you walk with me?"

I answered, "I would be honored." I squeezed her hand and was surprised how cold it was, despite the warm weather and the fact that she was wearing a long-sleeved survivor t-shirt. Monica was 39 years old and half a head taller than me, but I still felt like I was standing beside an anxious little girl.

"I know I'm going to lose it. I just know I'm going to lose it," she said. I told her that crying was nothing to be ashamed of and asked how Dale was doing. (Dale was ahead of us with the other blue-shirted walkers.) She said that Dale was standing with two teachers whom they had met, but that he was probably going to lose it, too.

As we slowly approached the stage area, Monica and I linked elbows, and I did the same with the third pinkie in our row. With her free arm, Monica waved at the applauding, cheering crowd and called, "Thank you." She vacillated between smiling and wiping away tears. Repeatedly, she apologized for crying and, just as often, I reassured her that crying was okay. When we reached the entrance to the stage area, with its stunning backdrop of the Capitol a few blocks away, the three of us unlinked our elbows and held hands, preparing to raise our arms for the victory walk. We waited for our cue from Nancy Mercurio, national spokesperson for the Breast Cancer 3-Day, who was at the microphone.

Nancy had already introduced the blue-shirted walkers and the white-shirted volunteer crews. Each group had surged into the stage area to upbeat music, cheers, and applause. Now it was time for the last group—the survivors—to enter. The music shifted to a reflective tone, and Nancy was no longer a cheerleader for tired walkers and volunteers. Instead, she was the daughter of a woman who had lost a nine-year battle with breast cancer.

Nancy described the breast cancer survivors as being extraordinarily committed to finding a cure for breast cancer. Their decision to walk or volunteer in the 3-Day indicated that surviving their personal battle with cancer "was not enough." The music abruptly shifted. It was time for our victory walk.

By the time Nancy finished the introduction, Monica was sobbing. I wrapped my arms around her waist and mumbled, "It's okay, Sugar." ("Sugar" is one of my pet names for my young nieces, my fiancé's young children, and even for my grown children.) It was then that I began to cry, too. After all, I was standing beside a young woman who would probably not live to see her young sons become adults.

When I had learned that Monica had Stage IV breast cancer, my first reaction was denial. Here she is, I had thought, tanned skin, sun-bleached hair, sturdy, laughing, holding hands with her husband, walking briskly. It just can't be true that she has advanced disease. It just *can't be true*, I had wanted to scream. At times during their story, I had wanted to stop my ears, particularly when I realized the rawness of their emotions— her fear and dread; his anger, sadness, frustration, and guilt. I soon realized, though, that to shy away from what she and her husband and two young sons were facing would be shirking my obligation to gather and shape stories. Still, it was difficult to continue listening (and not find a way to change the subject) when she said she hoped to survive long enough for her death not to be disastrous for her sons.

We raised our hands above our heads and strode forward. As we passed the other walkers, I glimpsed Dale Cooper, with his defiant Mohawk haircut and earrings and his chiseled, clenched jaw. He was crying, too.

Near the end of Closing Ceremonies, a group of five breast cancer survivors, holding hands in a circle, moved toward the stage. They surrounded a man carrying a sky-blue flag. Three days before, at Opening Ceremonies, the same group of breast cancer survivors, holding hands in a circle, had moved toward the stage. At Opening Ceremonies, the circle had been empty. The circle's emptiness symbolized the absence of family members and friends who had died. The empty circle symbolized sorrow. But, as Nancy Mercurio pointed out, at Closing Ceremonies the circle was no longer empty. Now it held a blue flag—an empty blue flag. Using the empty flag as a departure point— as a clean slate—Nancy urged each of us to develop our own "vision of a world without breast cancer ... not ordered by the limits of the past, but wide open to the wildest of dreams."

I doubt if there was a single listener who wasn't moved by the closing words: "For three days, we have been saying, 'We walk because we believe.' And today, let us renew our promise together, shouting to the tired ears of the world: 'We will never give up. We believe in a world without breast cancer, and *we will never give up.*'"

As the music roared to an upbeat song, I hugged Monica goodbye and told her to take care of herself. She flashed one of her best smiles and said, "Maybe I'll see you at next year's walk." Our eyes met and I smiled back. I paused before I answered, "I hope so, Sugar." I turned quickly because I didn't want her to see me cry again.

I was walking alone during the afternoon of Day 2 when Monica and Dale passed me on a hill. I had noticed them earlier—a handsome young couple, tall and athletic—because they were holding hands as they walked. As they passed me, Monica said, "So you're a survivor, too?" We started chatting; soon, they were sharing their story.

Monica was 35 years old when her husband, Dale, discovered a lump in her breast. Because of her age, Monica was not initially concerned about it. "I kind of put it off, put it off. I kept thinking it was a cyst. I had been to the doctor at one point [approximately two years before the mass was discovered], and she had said I had very fibrous breasts from caffeine. So, I thought, It's just caffeine, but it kept getting bigger and bigger."

Monica's primary care physician ordered first a mammogram, then a magnification mammogram, and finally an ultrasound. A "magnification mammogram" is just what it sounds like. An area that is worrisome by standard mammography technique is selectively examined ("coned down on"). This imaging study is particularly useful for evaluation of tiny calcifications that might signify ductal carcinoma *in situ* (DCIS).

Monica's mother was in the examination room with her during the ultrasound. "I remember my mom sitting at the end of the bed [examining table], and I mouthed to her, 'How many?' and she just kept holding up fingers. It turned out that I had 10 tumors between 0.8 and 2.8 cm, and I had calcifications everywhere. My breasts looked like they were full of sand."

The following day, Monica and Dale Cooper met with a surgeon. "She said, 'You're going to have to have a mastectomy,' and I remember Dale said, 'What? My wife was perfectly fine yesterday.' It kind of threw our lives into total turmoil. I didn't even have surgery first. I went in the next week and got a mediport and started chemo the next day. I started out with Adriamycin® and Cytoxan®—four cycles—then we stopped for about three weeks. The day of the Race for the Cure®—which I had honestly done every year for 11 or 12 years; it was the only time I missed it—was the morning of my surgery. Modified radical [mastectomy] with nodes. Five nodes positive. Then four cycles of Taxol®. Radiation, 40 sessions. Tamoxifen." Monica spoke perfunctorily, as if she had often repeated her medical history, or as if she were reciting a stranger's medical history.

As opposed to *adjuvant* chemotherapy, which is given after surgery, *neoadjuvant* chemotherapy is given prior to surgery. Monica received both. Neoadjuvant chemotherapy is most commonly used as a means to shrink the primary tumor in a patient with locally advanced disease. Certain patients who would otherwise have required a mastectomy become candidates for breast conservation treatment, and patients with large, initially unresectable tumors become candidates for resection. Neoadjuvant chemotherapy is also commonly used for inflammatory breast carcinoma, which will be mentioned in Chapter 7 about San Diego.

For about a year and a half after Monica completed chemotherapy, her follow-up studies indicated that she was free of disease, and she was beginning to reclaim the life of a physically active, working mom. Then, while she was training for a triathlon, she fell off her bicycle and hurt her left shoulder. The injury seemed to heal, but a short time later, when she was at the water park with her sons, she fractured her coracoid process (a part of the shoulder blade, or scapula, that overhangs the shoulder joint) while going down a water slide. A routine x-ray ("plain film") was suspicious for a "pathologic fracture."

"Pathologic" designates a subset of fractures that occurs at places where the bone has been weakened or thinned (or even completely replaced) by a tumor or some other disease process. Such fractures can result from relatively minor trauma, such as a bump while going down a water slide. They can even occur spontaneously.

A subsequent bone scan and magnetic resonance imaging (MRI)—two special types of imaging studies—confirmed that Monica's fracture was due to metastatic carcinoma. These tests also detected metastatic carcinoma in one of her ribs. Monica and Dale learned the results of the imaging studies on July 28, 2003. Monica's doctor reached them on their cell phone. They were at the beach with their sons.

Monica, Dale, and Monica's mother met with the medical oncologist the following week. Monica said, "When we were in before, she [the oncologist] was always very perky, very happy. She's young, in her 40s. She's awesome and is well known as the golden girl around here as far as oncology. When we went in for the first appointment after my recurrence, she came into the room and said, 'Well, Monica, it's spread. You're in a different stage now. It changes everything. Metastatic cancer is so different.' Then she said, 'I have one thing to tell you. Focus on your quality of life.'

"I thought, Quality of life? What does she mean, quality of life? So I pondered that for a long time. I actually called her back later and said that I needed to see her again. Since Dale and my mom had been there, I don't think she wanted to go into too much detail. I remember when I went back in to see her, I said, 'I need to ask you this. It's just driving me crazy. What do you mean?'

"She said, 'Monica, I can't tell you for sure. The way things are today, I could tell you that you might live two years. I could tell you that you might live five or 10 years. Realistically, right now I don't have any patients who have lived longer than 10 years. But,' she said, 'things are always changing, and you may be the one that lives 20 years.' She said, 'I'm being honest with you. You're very young and your cancer is very aggressive.'"

Monica glanced at Dale, but he was staring straight ahead, jaw set. She slipped her hand into his hand and paused. He nodded and tried to smile at her. She continued. "I went through a stage where I mourned. I was very angry. I didn't leave the house. I wanted to be around my kids all the time. I got into my yard work. I got into making little bracelets and things. I sort of shut everything down. I think I needed to mourn myself, but then, I thought, I can't do this. I started doing a lot of different things and trying to be real active. Now, I'm good, but I know, realistically, that it's never going to go away."

Monica received external beam radiation treatment to the metastases in her rib and her right shoulder, and began receiving intravenous infusions of Aredia® (pamidronate disodium) every three weeks. This pharmaceutical agent is a powerful aminobiphosphonate. It helps stabilize the remaining bone at metastatic sites by inhibiting bony resorption (loss) that is caused by the tumor. Because of the risk of kidney damage, Aredia® must be infused very slowly. Another newer agent, Zometa® (zoledronic acid, also an aminobiphosphonate), works similarly to Aredia®. Zometa® has the advantage of not taking as long for the infusion process (15 minutes as opposed to two hours for Aredia®); however, it, too, can cause kidney damage, and this complication must be carefully monitored.

Both Aredia® and Zometa® also help with the treatment of hyper-calcemia of malignancy—the increased level of calcium in the blood, which sometimes results from metastatic disease or from tumors that destroy bony tissue. Lastly, some studies have examined the usefulness of these drugs for preventing osteoporosis among breast cancer survivors, which is associated with early menopause, chemotherapy, and aromatase inhibitors. In Europe, an oral aminobiphosphonate has been approved, so this may be the next agent that is introduced in the United States.

Monica said, "I am what is called 'stable.' I still have lots of cancer in my shoulder and my rib still lights up, but it has been irradiated. Every three weeks until ..." Monica paused briefly, then corrected herself, "—forever—I will be getting the bone density medicine. It seems to be helping. I'm able to do things. I haven't broken anything else, knock on wood." She tapped her head. "Every three months I go for CAT [computerized axial tomography] scans, bone scans, and we alternate PET [positron emission tomography] scans. There are no guarantees." Monica smiled and shrugged. "She [the medical oncologist] said, 'Live your life to the fullest,' which I have."

Monica participated in her first 3-Day walk in 2003, a few months before she learned that she had metastatic (Stage IV) cancer. Dale did not participate with her in 2003 but, about the 2004 walk, he said, "This is my first walk. I'm such an idiot for not doing it the first time. If I'd done this the first time, I think I would have understood. This walk, for me, has been outstanding. It just brings everything into focus."

Later during our conversation, when Monica had stepped away to answer her cell phone, Dale said, "Unfortunately, it has taken me three years to come to terms with this ... It's crazy. Both of us are doing the therapy thing. I'm trying to deal with it on my terms. She's trying to deal with it on her terms. It's been very traumatic. I've been running away for two years, and she's been putting up with crap. Until you're in that position, you can't imagine. It has the potential to wipe out our whole family. It requires a whole new life strategy. Monica is *39*. Cancer is an *old lady* disease. We've come very close to splitting up because of how I've been dealing with it, how she's been dealing with it. For me, it's been either denial or betrayal—either it doesn't exist or she's going to die, and I'm going to move forward with my life. Just recently, we've gotten back together. Regardless of what happens, we have to stay together. We have no other options."

Dale continued. "We both had careers, rolling in the dough, and then all of a sudden ..." His voice trailed off and he shook his head. He continued, his voice becoming husky. "You realize what you can lose in an instant. Ironically, her last chemo was on 9/11. She was in downtown D.C. on a sales call when the attacks happened ... She was trying to make it to chemo and was right there in front of the White House.

She was on her cell phone and said, 'Oh, look. There are rockets on top of the White House.' Somehow we made it to chemo. We were sitting there, watching stuff unfold on TV, and she had a needle in her arm. It was wild. We realized how quickly you could lose something. Not to be spiteful, but while watching those people on TV, I felt like saying, 'Now you get it. Now you know how it feels.'"

Monica said that her greatest concern was for their sons, Joseph and James (Joey and Jamie). "My doctor told me last July that I qualify for disability and asked me why I was working. At first, I said that I didn't want to give up my life, but then in April [2004], I thought, My kids are my life. Why am I working? So I retired. This has been a good summer. We've gone to the beach. We're just enjoying life ... The part that's hard for me is the uncertainty, especially when I think about my kids. I don't ever want to be away from them. That's why I retired. I told Dale that if anything were to ever happen to me, I want them to remember me."

Monica Cooper may have been easy to find in the crowd because of her height, but Katey Arnold, 30, stood out because of her wide-brimmed straw hat. Katey was a slender young woman who didn't look much older than my college-aged daughter Jessica. Her straw hat may have caught my attention, but it was the compression sleeve, which she was wearing on her arm, that startled me. A compression sleeve meant that she was a breast cancer survivor.

Some women who have been treated for breast cancer develop problems with lymphedema of the arm or breast. This is a chronic or intermittent swelling due to pooling of lymphatic fluid in tissue, which can cause heaviness, redness, and pain in the affected area. It happens most often after removal of five or more lymph nodes from the axilla (armpit), but it can also occur after multifield irradiation of the axilla. Breast lymphedema most often occurs after there has been surgery in the upper outer quadrant of the breast and usually responds well to manual lymphatic drainage (MLD) by a trained physical therapist.

Arm lymphedema, in contrast, can be a major problem, and there is no cure. In fact, it can worsen over time. MLD is also helpful for arm lymphedema, but more severe lymphedema also requires consistent use of a compression sleeve, like the one that Katey was wearing. Women with mild arm lymphedema sometimes choose to wear the compression sleeve (which can be uncomfortable and restrict mobility) only when they are in high-risk situations, like flying on an airplane or engaging in vigorous physical activity—like walking 60 miles, maybe?

Katey Arnold was 27 years old and attending law school when she was diagnosed with breast cancer. "When I was diagnosed [in 2001], there really wasn't very much in my hometown, so I just started searching for information on the Internet. I was fortunate to come across the Web site for the Young Survival Coalition® (YSC) early on and to meet some really great people. It's terrible for anybody to go through what I did, but it makes it a lot easier when there are people to talk to who have been there, and who can kind of say, 'Oh, yeah, this will happen' and 'That will happen' and 'Here's what I did.' It made it a whole lot easier for me; then I can do the same thing for people that come after me."

YSC (www.youngsurvival.org) was formed in 1998 by three young breast cancer survivors who, according to the organization's Web site, were "discouraged by the lack of information and resources available to young women, and concerned about the under-representation of young women in breast cancer studies." The organization now has thousands of survivors and supporters, with the motto, "Action, Advocacy, Awareness." Evidently the efforts of YSC (and like-minded people) are successful, because the number of published articles in the medical literature that specifically addresses the concerns of women of child-bearing age with breast cancer has quadrupled since 1998. And, as Katey stressed—and like the Web site says—"The YSC also serves as a point of contact for young women living with breast cancer." For Katey, the YSC was a beacon.

"I was 27 when I was diagnosed, but there are a lot of people in the YSC who were much younger than I was when they were diagnosed—in their early 20s. It's so disheartening, but most of them are doing really well, so there are stories of hope and inspiration, too. [They] are a very strong reason to continue doing things like this [the 3-Day walk].

"I am two years out from treatment, three years out from diagnosis. They took 18 lymph nodes when I had my mastectomy. My tumor was really, really large. Fortunately, the axillary lymph nodes were all clear. When I went in for the biopsy, they went on ahead and did the mastectomy; then I had chemo; then radiation; then chemo again. Because of my age, they wanted to be as aggressive as possible. It was not the best year of my life. I'm very glad that it's over with."

Katey Arnold did not withdraw from law school during her treatment; instead, she continued with her classes. "I wasn't living in the same town as my parents, and they came up for every single treatment—to be there with me—which really made a huge difference. I know it was really, really hard on them. I had the genetic testing [for *BRCA1* and *BRCA2* mutations] and I was negative. I was really relieved because I was worried about my mom. I didn't want her to have to go through this … Mother handled it like a champ. She's here cheering."

Katey's walking partner was her childhood friend, Jennifer King. This was their second 3-Day walk, the first being in Atlanta in 2003. Katey walked because she was a breast cancer survivor and an activist; Jennifer walked because "That's what a friend does." Jennifer and Katey have been friends since meeting in elementary school in Tuscaloosa, Alabama. They remained friends through junior high and high school, and kept in touch during their college years when Katey left Alabama to study mathematics and philosophy at the University of North Carolina at Chapel Hill and Jennifer stayed in Tuscaloosa to study nursing at the University of Alabama.

Their life trajectories diverged for a few years after college. Katey taught school for two years, then "got bored and went to law school." Meanwhile, Jennifer got married, finished nursing school, and obtained a master's degree as a nurse practitioner. She and her husband then joined the Peace Corps.

Jennifer said, "My husband was a journalist, and he hated it. I had just finished my first master's program, and I didn't know what I wanted to do with it. We hadn't bought a house yet, and we weren't sure where we were going to live. We had no real debt—which was a plus for the Peace Corps, because you don't really get paid—when he said he'd like to do it. I said 'Okay, let's try it.' So we did.

"It was the most incredible experience, outside of these two 3-Day walks, truly. These have been the three best experiences of my life— Peace Corps and doing the two 3-Day walks with Katey." She and Katey looked at each other and smiled. "Nothing compares to it ... A lot of people go into the Peace Corps thinking they are going to change the world, save people. The reality is that they did way more for us than we could ever imagine doing for them ... The really tough part was being pulled out [of Uzbekistan] unexpectedly and how 9/11 played into it— the drama of 9/11 in America versus the drama of 9/11 very far removed from it.

"I came home the week Katey had her mastectomy. I called her up one day and said, 'What have you been up to?' She said, 'Well, I had a mastectomy.' I couldn't talk." Katey and Jennifer looked at each other and giggled. Jennifer continued. "I didn't even know about it. I was in hiding—quarantined away for a while. As soon as I could, I got right down there."

Paralleling Katey's passionate advocacy for young breast cancer survivors is Jennifer's passionate advocacy for her women patients. To accomplish this, she returned to school for additional training. "I'm back in school getting my post-master's as a primary care nurse practitioner, which I really, really love, because I get to do women's exams. That's my favorite thing, being an advocate for women. Starting right here." She linked elbows with her longtime friend, and they laughed again.

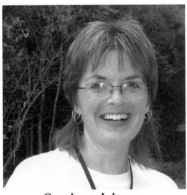

Carolynn Johnson

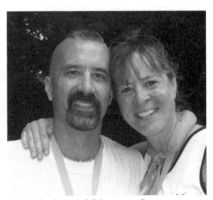

Dale and Monica Cooper

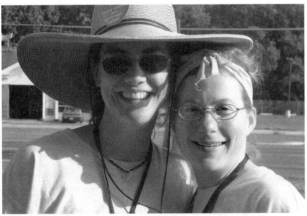

Katey Arnold and Jennifer King

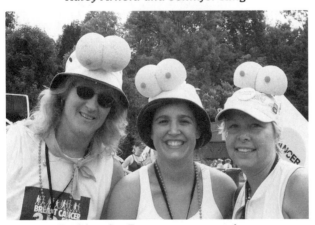

Buddies for Breasts team members

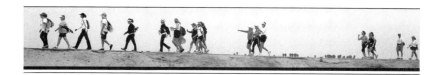

Chapter 4

Michigan

August 20, August 21, and August 22, 2004

Ask a Michigan resident where they live and they'll raise their right hand with the thumb extended and fingers together and point to a place on their palm or, less often, on their thumb or on one of their fingers. This is what they do for the Lower Peninsula. If, on the other hand (literally), they are talking about the Upper Peninsula, they'll show you the back of their left hand, with the index, middle, and ring finger together and the thumb and pinkie extended. This is their geographic shorthand for the relatively solid chunks of a state that are otherwise inundated. I say "relatively solid" because Michigan is defined by great big lakes and strewn with 11,000 crumbs of water.

I asked one particularly friendly woman to show me (on her hand) where Battle Creek was located. She indicated a spot about an inch below the middle of her palm and smiled. "So you want to know where all your cereal comes from, right?"

"No," I said. "Actually, I was born in Battle Creek."

She looked puzzled and, after pausing, she said, "But you didn't grow up in Michigan, did you?" (It was probably my drawl that tipped her off.)

The fact I wasn't born in Texas has dogged me since the first day of third grade. Back then, our family lived in Kermit—a West Texas oil boom town with a population of 15,000, roughly twice what it had been a decade before. If you knew Texas geography but couldn't pinpoint Kermit, I would tell you, "Kermit is 50 miles due west of Odessa," and you'd nod your head, "Oh, sure. Got it." If you didn't know the state, I would say, "You've heard of the Texas Panhandle, at the top of the state? Well, Kermit is in that little armpit where it cradles the southeastern corner of New Mexico." You'd probably squint your eyes a little, visualizing Texas's elbows and knees, and nod, "Oh, okay. Sure. Got it." What you might not appreciate is the part about the armpit. (People who don't know any better call that part of Texas "the armpit" to be disparaging.)

Back to third grade in Kermit. Our teacher, Mrs. Parsons, had us take turns telling what town we lived in when we were a little-bitty-baby. (As the county seat, Kermit's hospital provided obstetrical support for the armpit—thus, Mrs. Parsons's distinction between where we were *born* and where we actually *lived*.) Most of the places that my classmates named were within about a 50-mile radius: Midland, Odessa, Monahans, Andrews, Crane, Wink, and Notrees (pronounced "no trees," which hints at Kermit's location at the northeastern corner of the Chihuahuan Desert). A few of my classmates had even lived in *big* cities, *far* away, such as Amarillo, Lubbock, and El Paso.

When it was my turn, I said, "Battle Creek, Michigan."

Mrs. Parsons smiled—to this day, I don't think she meant to be unkind—and said, "Well, we have ourselves a little Yankee." Most of the class probably didn't understand the significance of being called a "Yankee," and if my mother hadn't grown up in Georgia, with most of her family still living there, I probably wouldn't have either. However, I had been led to believe by my mother's older brothers that being a Yankee was nearly as reprehensible as being a cockroach. In fact, I rarely heard them say "Yankee" without a qualifying "damn." (My mother's people are Church of Christ and seldom use profanity; however, they make exceptions when talking about Yankees.)

"No, ma'am," I said. "I'm not a Yankee!" And I started to cry.

That night, I told my native Texan father what had happened and asked him if I was a Yankee. He said, "Oh, for crying out loud. Of course not." He explained that, when I was born, he was stationed at Percy Jones Army Hospital in Battle Creek and, by the time I was six months old, we were back in Texas. "Besides," he said, "people could care less where you're born, just as long as you're smart and tactful." I promptly looked up "tactful" in the dictionary and decided that Mrs. Parsons hadn't been very tactful when she called me a Yankee.

I recovered from being called a Yankee and (pretty much) overcame not being a native Texan—at least I hardly ever cried about it again. When our family left Kermit and moved to Austin, my world widened. I realized, among other things, the absurdity of stereotyping Yankees. The cheery companion of Yankee contempt is, of course, southern pride or, more particularly, Texas boosterism, which, taken to an extreme, is obnoxious. I don't think I've ever stood accused of that, but I do admit a moderate fondness for what some call the "Texas mystique"—warts, wastefulness, and some undeniable wickedness notwithstanding. I doubt I could get used to living anywhere else.

In spite of what some of my fellow Texans claim, however, ours is not the only beautiful state. Michigan is beautiful, too, at least in the suburbs west and northwest of Detroit—beginning in Ypsilanti and ending in Orchard Lake—where we walked. *Absolutely beautiful.* It's not that I expected dingy factories with choking fumes pouring out of smokestacks beside heaps of discarded tires, but I was still astonished by the Michigan countryside. For the first time in my life, I found myself bragging that I was born in Battle Creek. To add a little twist to the situation, my 52nd birthday was during the Michigan walk on August 21. I was born in 1952 and I was back again in my birth state for the first time in nearly 52 years. What a chance circumstance.

———

Two chance circumstances had major impacts on Kim Clexton's life. The first was when she was in college and was stood up for a date. She was understandably furious. As a consolatory gesture, Kim's roommate invited Kim to join her and her boyfriend at his apartment to watch TV. Kim described what happened: "My roommate said, 'Come over to Mark's. We're just going to watch a movie.' I said, 'Well, *there's* the remedy for getting stood up. I'll go over and be a third wheel.' Then my roommate said, 'It's not like that.' At first, I wasn't going to go, but I didn't want to sit there and feel sorry for myself. Frankly, I didn't want to sit around and wonder if this guy was going to call me after all. So I went over there."

The roommate's boyfriend shared an apartment with a man named John Clexton, whom Kim had never met before. In fact, she was only dimly aware that Mark even had an apartment-mate. When she arrived, John was fixing dinner for himself. "I'll never forget this. John was making pasta and boxed mashed potatoes. Spaghetti noodles. He had no sauce. He was going to butter the noodles. That's what he had in his cupboard at the time and that was what he was making for dinner. When you think about the whole low-carb thing. Omigod! We started talking and flirting and talking some more and flirting some more. We talked until four o'clock in the morning ... I knew almost immediately." If Kim hadn't been stood up, she might never have met her future husband.

Another chance circumstance resulted in a diagnosis of breast cancer in 2002 at age 33. Kim had experienced a few mild episodes of *left*-sided bloody nipple discharge about two weeks before she was scheduled for her annual pap smear. Eight months before, when Kim and John's third child was born, Kim had attempted to breastfeed their newborn daughter; however, the baby developed thrush (candidiasis of the tongue), which secondarily infected Kim's nipple. She described the discomfort as "the old cat on the ceiling feeling" and she was forced to switch to bottle feedings. When she developed the tiny bit of bleeding from her left nipple, she attributed it to her previous infection and didn't give it much thought, despite the six-month hiatus.

By the time Kim had an appointment for her annual pap smear, it had been two months since the last episode of bleeding. As an "oh-by-the-way," Kim mentioned the bleeding to her gynecologist. The doctor thought it was odd but, since no masses were palpable, she agreed with Kim's self-diagnosis of some residual infection of one of the major lactiferous (milk-conveying) ducts. All the same, she wisely (and, serendipitously, it turned out) ordered a mammogram to evaluate Kim's left-sided nipple discharge.

After the mammogram, Kim was asked to remain in the waiting room. "While I was in the waiting room, the [radiology] tech came out and asked, 'Which breast was it that you said you had a discharge from?' and I said my left. And she said, 'Interesting.' I said, 'What does that mean, *interesting?*'" Kim squinted her eyes and waggled her head.

"She left and came back and said they saw a shadow in the *right* breast, and they wanted to send me for an ultrasound. The nice thing was that I could go right away. Everyone I have talked to since then has said that they had their mammogram, but their ultrasound was a week later. So I went and had my ultrasound. They told me, 'Your doctor will have the results in five days.'

"I didn't feel anything [in the right breast], so I wasn't terribly concerned ... Because of the episode of bleeding from the left nipple, they eventually did do an ultrasound on the left—just to make sure—but there was absolutely nothing there ... At one time, they even talked about doing nipple ductography, but the nipple bleeding has never happened since."

Also called "galactography," ductography is sometimes done when a woman (or man) experiences nipple discharge. The procedure involves using a blunt-ended needle to inject radiopaque contrast fluid into the nipple duct that the discharge is coming from, then doing mammograms to evaluate the duct system.

Kim continued. "I couldn't wait five days, so I started calling the doctor's office. The second time I called, I got a nurse, and she said, 'We understand your concern. You have a cyst. It's a fairly large cyst, so it will have to have a needle drainage. You will need to see a surgeon. Go to your primary care physician to get a referral.'

"I said, 'Okay.' She was using all these terms that I didn't understand. 'So, bottom line,' I said, 'we're not talking about cancer, right?'

"'Oh, no, no, no, it's not cancer,' she said.

"It was right before Halloween and Christmas—with all the stuff going on with small kids—and luckily, I didn't say, 'I can deal with this later.' I went to see my primary care physician and got a referral to a surgeon two weeks later. I was starting to get a little nervous, so I asked him, 'Can you just explain to me what they're seeing on the ultrasound that they're sure it's not cancer?'

"There was a shocked look on his face. He said, 'Are we ruling out cancer? All of your history—your risk factors—point to no cancer, but I wouldn't look at this mass on the ultrasound and tell anyone with any kind of certainty that it's not cancer, just because there's a solid edge. It's not a clear-cut cyst.'"

Kim was referred to a general surgeon for aspiration of the "cyst" (which was nondiagnostic) and later an excisional breast biopsy. About a week after the surgery, she and her husband, John, arrived at the surgeon's office for a 4:30 PM appointment. When she was summoned to an exam room, John stayed behind in the waiting room; however, after a few minutes, he came into the exam room. Kim asked him what he was doing there, and he answered that the nurse had told him that he should be in the exam room with her. Kim's immediate response was, "Omigod, I've got cancer."

Despite John's attempts to reassure her, Kim's anxiety intensified as she waited. The surgeon proceeded to see every other patient—even those who had arrived after Kim—before coming to Kim's exam room. "I could hear him basically clearing out the office. I was stunned, thinking, Maybe I don't. Maybe I don't. Maybe I'm assuming these things. Finally he came in and, sure enough, said, 'Come back into my office.'

"He's a very nice guy but was totally unprofessional about breaking the news to me. He described what the next year would be like, the whole scenario. He didn't hold back anything. It was too much information, and not all of it was entirely accurate. The other thing that he did— and I appreciate that he was trying to make me feel better—was to tell me that he had only one testicle, and that I had a loving guy as my husband, and it really wasn't going to be a big deal if I had to have a mastectomy. Okay, I was thinking, that's more than I needed to know about you."

Kim shook her head and laughed. "John and I sort of looked at each other and went, *all right* ..." Kim widened her eyes and grimaced. "But it was good, because it held me over until I got to the car. When he was talking about his testicle, I was too caught up in the absurdity of the situation. I kept thinking, You have *what*? I couldn't get the image out of my brain." Kim covered her eyes with her hands and laughed again.

Before she left the surgeon's office that afternoon, she had already decided that the first thing she was going to do was find a surgeon who specialized in breast surgery. "When the biopsy results came back—it was essentially a lumpectomy—the edges weren't clean, so we weren't certain that he had gotten it all. He [the surgeon] said, 'I can go back in, and I can make sure I can get clean margins, or we can do a mastectomy. Just let me know when you're ready.' I was walking out thinking, I'm not coming back here."

Kim's conclusion that she "needed to find a breast doctor" may have been intuitive; however, her intuition was later supported by a retrospective study of five-year survival rates among 29,666 breast cancer patients in Los Angeles County. The study was conducted by researchers at the Keck School of Medicine (at the University of Southern California at Los Angeles), with results published in a 2003 article in *Annals of Surgical Oncology*: "Multivariate analysis indicated that type of surgeon was an independent predictor of survival (relative risk, .77), as were both hospital and surgeon case volume." This meant that breast cancer patients treated by cancer surgeons had a 33% reduction in the risk of death at five years.

Elizabeth Naftalis, M.D., Assistant Professor of Surgery, UT Southwestern Center for Breast Care, commented on this study in a 2004 article in *Breast Diseases: A Year Book® Quarterly:* "This article from the Keck School of Medicine is quite timely, as we have just this year begun a national breast fellowship match program. The Society of Surgical Oncology, the American Society of Breast Surgeons, and American Society of Breast Disease have all orchestrated this process, and the Susan G. Komen Breast Cancer Foundation was instrumental in helping establish the guidelines for this program. The importance of specialty training is once again enforced by this excellent, large study."

Kim didn't need the results from a large study to initiate what she called her "little breast cancer interviews." She, John, and her Aunt Geraldine, a nurse who worked at a local transplant hospital, talked to health care providers at the Van Elslander Cancer Center of St. John Hospital (Grosse Pointe Woods, Michigan) and the Barbara Ann Karmanos Cancer Institute (Detroit). Among the features of the Van Elslander Cancer Center that she liked best was the policy of assigning a nurse navigator to every new cancer patient. The nurse navigator introduced Kim to the team of doctors who would be involved with her care: the surgeon, the medical oncologist, and the radiation oncologist.

It was during this process that Kim began to have some doubts. "The oncologist was a very young, very nice guy. He had a pager and a cell phone going at all times—always answering it—and he was very distracted. He immediately started talking about clinical trials. Not that I'm not open to clinical trails, but I wanted to tell him, 'You're supposed to be talking to me about standard of care.'

"I went to Karmanos and met a surgeon named David Bauwman, who is a wonderful, huge teddy of a guy with a lot of hair on his face, who really made me feel very comfortable, and who answered all my questions. He was reassuring and gave me his home phone number and said, 'If you come up with any questions, call me.' The only down side— which we found out later—is that the reason he gave his home phone number is that it is almost impossible to reach anyone to answer any questions. None of his nurses are instructed to answer even simple questions.

"I later met another surgeon at St. John—one recommended by several other women. I had very high expectations of her. I've met her again since then, and she's a very nice woman, but she completely overwhelmed me. First, we waited for 45 minutes to see her, then she came in and talked the life out of me. I thought, Whoa. Calm down. She hugged me and then had to step back and look at the chart to figure out what my name was. If she can't remember my first name, she shouldn't be hugging me just yet. It sort of turned me off. So I ended up at Karmanos and decided to go with Dr. Bauwman."

In contrast to the Van Elslander Cancer Center, at St. John Hospital, Kim was not scheduled to meet with her medical oncologist until after her surgery was accomplished. "The one negative thing when I made my decision to go with Karmanos versus the community hospital was that the community hospital seemed to do a much better job of caring for the patient by having the nurse navigator take care of all kinds of silly questions. Karmanos wasn't going to have me meet with the medical oncologist until after my mastectomy. Well, I needed to know if I needed flu shots—just silly things like that. Simple questions for which I didn't think I needed to call the doctor at home. Somebody should be able to answer questions, so I felt very strongly that I should be seeing my medical oncologist before the mastectomy. I knew he couldn't give me any definite answers until they had the pathology, but give me an idea of what could be ahead of me instead of just going through this mysterious process and then heading into another mysterious process. So I really pushed it and got in to see him.

"I was very lucky, though, because I had my aunt, who worked at the transplant center, with me. Friends of mine had parents who worked there and who knew people who knew people that got me connected, and I pushed it. There's a whole lot of people out there who don't have those connections or even know the questions they should be asking. Maybe they're even afraid of asking them."

During the interviews with potential surgeons, Kim reviewed treatment options. Based on the size of her tumor (1.2 cm) and the fact that her axillary lymph nodes were clinically negative, Kim might have been a candidate for breast conservation therapy (BCT), which is a lumpectomy or wide local excision, with a sentinel node biopsy, followed by radiation treatment. However, there were other factors to consider. First, both invasive carcinoma and ductal carcinoma *in situ* were present in the biopsy. Second, the tumor was high-grade (poorly differentiated), estrogen-receptor (ER) negative, and overexpressed *HER-2*. Lastly, Kim had given birth eight months before she was diagnosed with breast cancer.

Several excellent medical studies have examined the effect of childbirth on subsequent breast cancer diagnosis. One of the more recent was a prospective study involving 750 women less than 45 years old who had been diagnosed with invasive breast cancer within five years of giving birth. Their risk of death from breast cancer was compared to that of women with breast cancer who had never given birth, and the results were troubling: "Proximity of last childbirth to subsequent breast cancer diagnosis is a predictor of mortality independent of histopathological tumor characteristics. Clinicians should be aware that women diagnosed with breast cancer within a few years following childbirth may have a worse outcome than that suggested solely by the standard histopatho-logical prognostic factors of their cancer."

Kim ultimately underwent a modified radical mastectomy and low axillary node dissection, followed by adjuvant chemotherapy. She had hoped to undergo an immediate reconstruction and, early on, she saw a plastic surgeon at St. John. "The plastic surgeon was a really nice guy and had actually worked on my son's finger when he partially severed it, but he was really into the idea of the TRAM flap [transverse rectus abdominis myocutaneous flap reconstruction] and not really taking into account my [three previous] caesarean sections. 'Oh, you're going to look great. It's going to be fantastic.' He was very much into the cos-metic side of it.

"I finally got in to see a plastic surgeon through Karmanos, but not until after Christmas. I was waiting to talk to him before scheduling a mastectomy. He said, 'I don't want to do an immediate reconstruction. You're sort of at that weight limit, and you've had healing problems in the past with incisions from your caesareans. I don't want to delay your chemo at all. I don't think immediate reconstruction is a good decision.'

"I had it in my head that, if I did the immediate reconstruction, I would be able to deal with it better. First of all, to hear that I was too heavy to get an immediate reconstruction was not a very happy thing, and I had to adjust to the idea that I was going to have to live with a mastectomy scar and figure out all that, and then wait for the reconstruc-tion. I was also very concerned with inconveniencing people by having to care for the kids two different times. I would have been happy to get that recovery time shmushed in together. So I was sort of devastated at that point, but I got over it.

"That actually made it easier for me that he was the right guy. Even though I was disappointed, this guy actually cared about me as a cancer patient, not as a cosmetic patient. Since I did have healing issues with everything, it was the best decision I ever made, but hard to take at the time."

After her mastectomy and axillary dissection (nine nodes were nega-tive), Kim underwent four cycles of Adriamycin® and Cytoxan® and was scheduled to receive four cycles of Taxotere® (docetaxel); however, within a day after receiving her first (and, as it turned out, her last) infusion of Taxotere®, she developed intolerable shooting pains in her legs. Severe neurosensory symptoms (abnormal skin sensations, such as burning or prickling, and pain) occur in about 5% of patients who are treated with Taxotere®, requiring discontinuation of treatment. Kim was one of those patients.

Throughout chemotherapy treatment, she continued her part-time job as an academic advisor for students at a local college. After her sec-ond treatment, she lost her hair. "I wore a wig. I started wearing it in mid-March. In early June, I was pulling into the parking lot at work with a friend. I hadn't put on my wig yet because it was hot. Our other friend saw us and said to someone, 'Thank goodness. She's not wearing her wig. I want her to feel comfortable in her own skin.' By then, I had put on my wig and gone in to work, but I heard what she had said. I was already not wearing my wig when I wasn't at work, so then I thought that I want to be a positive role model so that people will know that young people can get breast cancer. That's when I decided that those students were just going to have to get over it … I think I needed the wig for a little while." Kim giggled. "Vanity!"

Kim decided to wait until after her children's summer vacation to have reconstructive surgery. "I had TRAM reconstruction in late September 2003. That was probably the hardest thing of all, but it was a positive thing in terms of my body and what it did for my self-image. Through all that stuff [the mastectomy and chemotherapy], I wasn't really frightened …" Kim wriggled her nose and looked at me over the top of her sunglasses. "Well, not any more than you would normally be if someone told you that you had cancer.

"I really wasn't terrified of the surgery until I got to the TRAM flap. I was worried about the anesthesia. I had had anesthesia for all my C-sections. The first one was an emergency and the next two were scheduled. I think it was because it was optional—elective surgery—and I thought I was tempting fate too much. It's a long surgery, so I was a little nervous—actually, quite nervous—when I started thinking about it. I couldn't put my finger on it, but I just felt like things could really get messed up." She sighed heavily, before adding, "Anyway, I had the TRAM and there were a few complications. I had some skin that didn't take and they had to fix that. I actually didn't get my nipple until May [2004] and I just had my tattoo. So now I'm a tatooed lady." Kim laughed and shimmied her shoulders.

Kim did not participate in any support groups, and she and her husband did not seek professional counseling. This decision was somewhat based on time constraints. After all, she was rearing three children and working part-time. "John was very supportive but I felt so bad for him. As the person fighting the cancer, you have a job to do. You have something to focus on. There was nothing active that John could do to fight the cancer. I think that's a very difficult position for anyone to be in, particularly someone who has never won that kind of battle in the past. He was very distressed. John's father died from a rare liver disease when he was in his 60s and his mother died in 1996 at age 61 of multiple myeloma [malignant overgrowth of bone marrow plasma cells] … Even though everything pointed to things being fine with me, he really didn't trust the outcome very much."

Kim and John may not have investigated professional help for themselves, but when Kim realized that their four-year-old son was having difficulty understanding what was happening, she sought guidance from a social worker at Karmanos Cancer Institute. "I was very disappointed. I was referred to her by someone who was a friend of hers. I told her that I had issues with my kids, and she said, 'Well, we have a group of kids. Maybe your oldest daughter could be part of it, but she's kind of on the young side.'

"My son probably needed the most information at his level. He didn't understand it. Molly, our older daughter, could at least intellectualize and deal with it. She may not have liked it and may have been upset about it, but at least she understood that Mommy was sick, Mommy was going to get better, that there would be a period of time that we would be fighting the disease, and they would have to put up with me being sick. My son didn't understand that and I didn't know how to explain it to him. So he was affected the most. Her [the social worker's] inability to answer that was most disappointing ... I always thought that a major cancer center would be better at that. Fundraising and specializing as much as they do, that should be a done deal."

I agreed with Kim. At the very least, she could have referred Kim to an excellent article by Paula K. Rauch, M.D. (e-mail: prach@partners.org), who is Chief of the Child Psychiatry Consultation Service at Massachusetts General Hospital. In the 2002 article that originally appeared in the *Journal of Clinical Oncology* entitled, "Parents With Cancer: Who's Looking After the Children?," Dr. Rauch and her coauthors offered guidelines for parents, including how to talk about illness to children.

For instance, Kim and John Clexton might have benefited from this specific suggestion: "Preschoolers weave logic and fantasy together to arrive at an idiosyncratic understanding of the events in the world. They are egocentric and thus cast themselves as the cause of the events affecting them. It is therefore important to remind children between the ages of 3 and 7 years that the parent's illness is not a result of anything the child thought or did." The article went on to suggest ways to handle common questions that children might ask and give instructions about how to prepare a child for a visit to see the hospitalized parent.

Dr. Rauch and her co-workers at the Massachusetts General Hospital Cancer Center developed a clinical program called PACT (Parenting at a Challenging Time). Dr. Rauch described the program to attendees of the 2004 San Antonio Breast Cancer Symposium. She said that, in her group's experience, a critical step for the afflicted families was "re-establishing a normal routine." Once again, Kim didn't need a medical study. She intuitively knew what was best for her family. "We just decided to fight the cancer, take care of the kids, and try to have somewhat of a normal life."

The Michigan 3-Day was Kim's first long-distance walk for breast cancer; however, she has been involved with the Susan G. Komen Foundation's signature event, Race for the Cure®, since her college days when she was a member of Zeta Tau Alpha. Since 1992, Zeta Tau

Alpha has devoted its philanthropic efforts to breast cancer education, awareness, and research. They also cosponsor the National Series Breast Cancer Survivor Recognition Program with RE/MAX (a global real estate system of offices) providing the pink t-shirts and caps for survivors and the "In Memory Of" and "In Celebration Of" back signs for race participants. Each year, over 5,000 Zetas volunteer over 50,000 hours at Race for the Cure® events across the country. Kim was one of those volunteers.

"We volunteered for Race for the Cure® when I was in college and then started doing it when it was at the Detroit Zoo and in 2003 at Comerico Park. I had always done it with a friend or my mom or whomever. Then, last year, I was a survivor. I could do it as a survivor. I went online and found out you could do teams, so we did a team. We had 28 members and raised over $500. This year, we had 38 members. All three of our kids were there, too. The youngest was in a stroller. The older two, who are five and eight years old, were just going to walk the 1-mile event, but they ended up walking the entire 5K route."

"Tough little kids," I commented.

"Oh, yeah. They've been through a lot. *We've* been through a lot, our whole family. We're good, though." Then Kim smiled and nodded, her eyes shining. "*Real* good."

Gale Colston, 48, and her husband, Tim, had much less difficulty explaining cancer to their 18-year-old son than the Clextons did with their small children. Gale, who was 38 years old when she was diagnosed, said, "I don't know if little Tim ever grasped the magnitude. At 18 years old, he was just going away to college at the University of Toledo, starting a new life, living on campus. He didn't live through it like some kids would. I don't think he ever realized the severity of it until maybe the last five years. Since then, he's grown up and matured. He hears about and e-mails other kids about their mothers who have gone through things. I just don't think that he realized at the time, which maybe wasn't all bad, because I didn't have to deal with that side of it.

"I think the hardest part at the time was that little Tim was going away. We had just been working our home as a bed-and-breakfast for about a year. I was still working full time. We were just doing a lot of things and wanting to do a lot more things. We thought, Why the hell did this happen now? We're having the time of our lives."

As is the experience of many young women, Gale's diagnosis was delayed because of her gynecologist's false sense of security about the palpable mass. This assumption was based on her age, negative family history, and negative mammogram. Fortunately, the wait-six-months-and-reevaluate approach is not as common now for young women with a palpable breast mass as it was 10 years ago, when Gale was diagnosed. She also did not have an ultrasound to evaluate the abnormal finding, which is another difference from current evaluation standards.

"The gynecologist was comfortable with the lump. They sent me for a mammogram and everybody was saying, 'It's fine, it's fine.' I think if we had waited six months the outcome wouldn't have been nearly as good ... You're feeling yourself 24 hours a day, seven days a week. It really hadn't changed a lot, but when I went back, I said, 'I'm not comfortable,' and she said, 'Well, let's go see a surgeon.' So she sent me over and I think he knew right then because the nipple had dropped a little at the corner on just the one side. I had never paid any attention to it. He did a needle biopsy—nothing. He said, 'We need to schedule you,' and within a week, he had me back at the hospital doing a biopsy.

"They did a modified radical with 14 nodes—zero positive—and the reconstruction immediately. My reconstruction surgeon was one of the first ones who was doing the TRAM flaps. I was one of the first 100 in Dayton ... It was pure luck that we got hooked up that way. I had no idea what was available. I often say that, when I woke up, I didn't deal with the loss that some girls have to go through. He didn't do the nipple and all of that until after chemo was finished ... I think the tattoo was the most important part to me because when you look, you see dark spots and you're fine with it. Before I had that, it didn't matter if it was sticking out or not; it wasn't finished."

Gale received six cycles of chemotherapy. Throughout her treatment, she continued to work as a sales rep for a supplier of medical gases, such as oxygen and nitrogen. "I had an awful time with treatment. I was sick the whole time. I was a trooper, though. I was still working. I would have my treatment on Wednesday afternoon and they didn't see me until the following Monday. I was still green when I came in, but I was there ... I never had any problems with any of my counts, and I never missed a treatment. In fact, a lot of girls had to come back a week later [delay their chemotherapy treatment for a week] because their counts were low. I didn't have to because my counts were always good."

In medical-speak, Gale did not require reduction in relative-dose intensity (RDI). Adjuvant chemotherapy side effects require reduction in the chemotherapy dose or treatment delays of greater than seven days in more than half of patients with early-stage breast cancer, according to a recent nationwide survey. The commonest cause was the one Gale mentioned: a decrease in the patient's white blood cell (neutrophile) count (WBC). Since a low WBC increases a patient's susceptibility and inability to fight infections, either the chemotherapy dose must be decreased or the treatment postponed until the WBC improves.

If it becomes necessary to reduce the RDI to less than 85% of standard reference doses, chemotherapy loses some of its effectiveness. In other words, patients are at an increased risk for recurrence or death. Fortunately, prophylaxis (or rescue) with a granulocyte colony-stimulating factor such as filgrastim (Neupogen®)—which was not available 10 years ago when Gale and her breast cancer sisters (and brothers) were receiving treatment—nudges the bone marrow into producing more neutrophiles. In most cases, this allows patients to continue treatments on schedule.

When she was 26 years old, Gale had a hysterectomy and a unilateral oophorectomy (one ovary removed). For several years prior to her breast cancer diagnosis, she had been taking low-dose Premarin® (hormone replacement therapy). "It seemed like one month you're fine, the next you're not. That's why I had been taking it for several years. Right before we found the lump, I had a cyst on the ovary that they left behind. They were treating me with megadoses of hormones, trying to get it to go down. I finished that in August [1994] and found the lump in September."

Gale's tumor was estrogen-receptor (ER) and progesterone-receptor (PR) positive. After she finished chemotherapy, she was placed on tamoxifen. "I think I was almost into menopause when I started tamoxifen, but after that [beginning adjuvant hormonal treatment] I was completely into menopause at age 39: the hot flashes, the skin difference, the memory. The thing that was most disappointing was the loss of sex drive. If I had been married to anyone else but Tim, it probably would have crushed our marriage. He is truly the best thing in my life, so I told my doctor, 'I don't know if I have 10 years or 100 years left, but I'm not living like this.' I stopped taking the tamoxifen.

"My doctor said, 'It's your choice, Gale,' and I said, 'That's exactly right. It's my choice.'" Gale pressed her lips together and nodded her head once, to punctuate what she told the doctor. "I know that, if something comes back, I will second-guess myself. I can still remember one of the days. I was just so exhausted." Gale began to cry, but then composed herself and apologized before continuing. "I was sitting on the porch while Tim was mowing the yard. We always do the yard together. I do the push mower and he does the regular mower. This was in the spring and I was so cold. I was all wrapped up and it was a beautiful day. I was sitting there on a lawn chair and I was thinking, If I stood up, I could probably walk in and get a drink of water. I didn't even have the strength to do that. That's when I decided that I wasn't going to live my life like that. I just couldn't do it, so I quit tamoxifen.

"I think the low point in our marriage came about three years after the diagnosis. I was to the point where I was saying, 'I've had enough.' I think part of it was that when you're 40 years old, your lives are changing. You start to think, Okay, here's where my friends are, and here's where I am, and here's where my career is. I think it was all part of the struggle. Did we need a marriage counselor? I didn't know what we needed. If I could fix it, I would. I think the part about the sex drive had something to do with it, too."

Gale and I talked about how disappointed we were about our diminished sex drives. Like me, Gale's sexuality had been a core part of her life before breast cancer and menopause. Hormone replacement therapy was, of course, not advisable for either of us, since our tumors were ER positive. That left us, like so many others, in a hormone-deprived desert. When I described my premenopausal sex drive as having been an ever-present sound track in my life—usually at a low but audible volume, although situationally at a very high volume—Gale laughed at my metaphor but agreed with the idea.

We talked about what I had read about sexuality after breast cancer. We discussed the various suggestions and concluded that the problem of diminished sex drive, particularly for the middle-aged breast cancer survivor, was much more complicated than most of our treating doctors realized. The loss of libido was also much more problematical than many realized.

Earnest, honest conversations with partners (assuming that he or she is understanding) can certainly help, and there are sex counselors, of course, but magical fixes—like a new position, a vaginal lubricant, a purchase from Victoria's Secret, or a sexy movie—can only *turn up* an existing volume. Such measures do little to *restore* the background music. Because they have worked well for me—and I was speaking as a woman, not as a physician—I shared these suggestions with Gale: Do exercises that improve both cardiovascular fitness and flexibility. Whatever it takes, get enough sleep, and focus on what attracted her to Tim in the first place.

At the last suggestion, Gale described how she and Tim met. She was 15 years old and Tim was 18 when they became friends. Gale was showing pleasure horses and Tim was working for his uncle, who was a horse trainer. "Tim got the horses ready. He wrapped legs and all that kind of stuff for his uncle. We were going along in the pleasure class— which was walk, trot, and canter—and my bridle broke. You can't dismount or it disqualifies you. Tim came running out with a new bridle. I was on the horse, but he had the equipment to make it go. My shining knight came with armor." Gale chuckled and pumped her fist. "He put the bridle on my horse and I loped off. From then on, we became great friends.

"He lived across town [in Dayton]—we're talking 45 minutes away from each other—and I didn't drive, so we would see each other in the summertime more than anything. We were always ..." Gale paused and smiled dreamily. "Not sweethearts, exactly, but always pretty chummy for years at the show ... He was at the University of Cincinatti and I was in high school. We had an awards banquet and I needed an escort, so I called him. That was probably our first formal date." They were married less than two years later, when she had just turned 19 and he was 21.

In 2004, Gale and Tim were participating in their fifth Breast Cancer 3-Day event (the first was in Chicago in 2000, then Atlanta in 2001, Michigan in 2002, and San Diego in 2003). Together, they have organized teams and raised money for Making Strides Against Breast Cancer® and Strides for Life®. For most events, Gale walked and Tim was a member of one of the support teams. His involvement in Gale's breast cancer advocacy was not surprising since she said that they "do everything together."

She said, "You've met him. He's a godsend. He's so strong. I think the coolest thing from the get-go was that *we* were going to fight. It was never a question. The two of us were in this together. I mean that's the reason we do all of this. I couldn't do it without him. I don't know if I'd want to. That's a scary thought, too."

As we parted, Gale hugged me and we thanked each other repeatedly for our heart-to-heart talk about postcancer sexuality. We agreed that it was a huge relief to know that other women had similar problems and that there were possible remedies. After smiling mischievously, her parting words were, "I may have to put a 'Do Not Disturb' sign on our tent tonight."

<hr>

Like Gale and Tim Colston, Patrick (Tony) and Sherrie Antoszewski participated in the last Michigan 3-Day, which was held May 31 through June 2, 2002. At the time of the 2002 walk, Sherrie was 29 years old and had recently had a wedge resection of her lung for removal of a single focus of metastatic breast cancer. When Tony Antoszewski, 31, and I talked in August 2004, Sherrie was enjoying her longest disease-free interval since her initial diagnosis of breast cancer at age 25 in 1998.

Tony and Sherrie met just after her 21st birthday and had been dating for several years when they decided to get married. Tony said, "We were engaged, and she thought she felt something in her breast, and she said, 'Will you feel this?' and I said, '*Gladly!*'

"My mom has fibrocystic breasts, so I thought, Lumpy boobs, fine. Let's get it checked out anyway. What does it hurt to find out that you've got fibrocystic breasts? It turned out not to be that easy. She had an ultrasound—they couldn't tell because her breasts were so dense. I said, 'I don't think you have anything to worry about, but you can't be too sure.' It was both us and the doctors wanting to be sure. My wife is persistent. We couldn't stop until we knew 'yes' or 'no' for sure.

"They couldn't get it with an ultrasound [-directed fine-needle aspiration] or with a needle biopsy, so they did a surgical biopsy. The surgeon came out into the waiting room and said, 'I've see this a thousand times, and you've got nothing to worry about.' Then they called Sherrie up later and said, 'Oh, we forgot to tell you. At any postop visit, you need to bring along a family member.' That didn't really feel good." Tony paused and shook his head, as if remembering that day. "What we both knew deep down inside, but couldn't admit to each other, was that she'd been diagnosed with something that we didn't really want to know about.

"The day we were told about the cancer, we left the surgeon's office and went straight to the oncologist's office. We filled out the paperwork, and he [the medical oncologist, Dr. Daniel Lehman from Great Lakes Cancer Management Specialists] said, 'I'm not going to candy-coat it. This has been the worst day in your life, so far. I'm just going to make it worse. You want me to treat you, I'm going to douse you with chemo and radiation, and it isn't going to be easy, but I'll take care of it.'

"This is a fairly young oncologist, probably in his mid-40s. I thought, This cat just got out of school, and he's going to take care of my wife? We liked him, but we got second and third opinions. We went to U of M [the University of Michigan], and they scared the hell out of us, honestly. They talked about bone marrow transplants. 'Oh, good,' they said, 'you've got a twin sister. She's going to be a match.' We left there scared. We felt worse than when we walked in. It was like *holy cow*. In the end, we decided to go with the guy who opened his doors and got us in and didn't candy-coat it.

"U of M was a great facility and they were thorough, but they were just so advanced. Maybe they didn't realize that they needed to take it step by step. You can only handle so much. Sure, it's good to know what *could* happen and what the next step *could* be, but the first time you see somebody, if it isn't as dire as it could possibly be—and, at that stage, my wife's situation wasn't that advanced—it would have been better if they didn't go into so much detail.

"First, she had the surgery—a lumpectomy—and some nodes were taken out. Three of 17 nodes were positive, I believe. My wife can give you the exact numbers. Then she had chemo and then we had the wedding."

As their wedding day approached, Sherrie was still bald and eyebrow-less from chemotherapy. At the bachelorette party, one of her bridesmaids presented Sherrie with a baseball cap with an attached wedding veil, which was put to good use the next day. "A wig is hot," Tony said, "and we had an August wedding. It was muggy. Halfway through the wedding, she slipped off her wig and put on her baseball cap with the veil. Sherrie said, 'This is me. This is who I am.' She is awesome." Tony smiled and pressed his lips together. He swallowed hard before adding, in a whisper, "Just *awesome*."

When asked if he ever had any second thoughts about getting married after he learned that his bride-to-be had breast cancer, Tony seemed a little confused by my question. "It wasn't her choice to get it, right? I chose her. She would have done the same thing if the shoe were on the other foot."

Following chemotherapy, Sherrie received adjuvant radiation treatment. During the last week of her radiation treatment, Tony and Sherrie conceived a child; however, they didn't know about the pregnancy for nearly four months. "Sherrie's doctors said she wasn't going to have children and that she was going to be, at least for a while, sterile. She didn't have a period and she didn't have a period, but she didn't have them during chemo and radiation, so there you go." Tony shrugged. "Sherrie was going in for one of her follow-up CAT scans of the abdomen and pelvis and a bone scan. With the dye and all, those things usually take a long time—like a couple of hours. She had it scheduled for the middle of the day. It was the first time I didn't go to a doctor's appointment with her. Well, with the bone scan, you have to have a pregnancy test beforehand, right? So they took one and they came back and said, 'Sherrie, your doctor is on the phone, and he needs to talk to you.' I love our doctor. He said, 'What did you go ahead and do now?' Sherrie said, 'Huh?,' and he said, 'You got pregnant.'

"She called me up at work and said, 'I don't know how to tell you this, but I can't have the test [bone scan]. I'm pregnant.' I'm like, 'You're *what*? I thought we had … oh, yeah, there was that one time.'" Tony rolled his eyes, smiled sheepishly, and nodded.

"Sherrie's doctors were saying that they didn't know how likely it was that this would be a healthy baby. They wanted to know if we wanted to talk about the options. Honestly, we talked about our options, and we were thinking that maybe …" Tony paused and shrugged, obviously preferring not to say the words "therapeutic abortion" out loud, "… *that* was what we needed to do. There were a lot of people saying a lot of things. We talked to a couple of doctors. We talked to the family a little bit. My wife's Lutheran and I'm Catholic. For a while there, what we heard was so negative that we were believing it. Then we said, 'You know what? We can take care of it. We can handle it.'

"By the time we got to the high-risk obstetrician's office—this was four weeks after finding out Sherrie was pregnant—our minds were made up the other way … We found out that everything *was* fine. He said, 'I can see no reason why you can't have a healthy, normal child.' Oh, what a great feeling!" Tony looked up at the sky and sighed. "When we heard she was fine, we were like, *cool*. Then, we found out it was a girl, which was really cool, too. We both wanted kids. We had names picked out, even before we were married. At one point, it was possible that we would never have any. We thought, Let's get healthy first, then we'll worry about someone else."

Tony and Sherrie's perfectly healthy daughter, Alexandra, was born 14 months after they were married. Shortly after the birth of her daughter, Sherrie was diagnosed with a second breast cancer in the opposite (contralateral) breast. She was 27 years old, and she said, "Enough of this." She underwent bilateral mastectomy with TRAM reconstruction followed by a second series of chemotherapy treatments.

Sherrie has a twin sister named Dawn. When Sherrie was first diagnosed with breast cancer, she asked her medical oncologist if breast cancer was something that Dawn needed to worry about. He answered that it was very important that Dawn be carefully followed. When Sherrie told the medical oncologist that her sister was a waitress, not married, and didn't have health insurance, this credit to the medical profession said, "If your sister needs care, I'll make sure she gets it."

Dawn had not had a mammogram at that time, but she finally decided to have one after Sherrie's first recurrence. Tony continued. "Dawn is a procrastinator by nature. They are twins, but so unlike one another. Dawn finally said, 'Okay, I really do have to check this out,' and it turned out to be positive. I think it was a good thing that she did, because her cancer was *HER-2* positive, more aggressive, more advanced, 12 of 18 nodes positive. Dawn said, 'Okay, just remove both breasts.' She decided to have tissue expanders put in. She was going to go for reconstruction—to have the implants put in—but she turned up pregnant. [Dawn had since gotten married.] So they put that off for awhile.

"She's on Herceptin® either every three or four weeks. My wife's was ER positive and *HER-2* negative. These are identical twins with completely different types of tumors, so there's no rhyme or reason. They are the first cases of breast cancer in their family. Maybe it's environmental, but their mother has lived in that house since before the kids were born. Neighborhood friends who grew up with them ... nothing." Tony shook his head. "Maybe God thought that they were the ones who could handle it. I don't know. I know my wife has it and she can handle it. She's a rock."

Shortly before Tony and Sherrie walked in the 2002 Michigan Breast Cancer 3-Day, Sherrie was diagnosed with metastatic disease in her lung. This meant, of course, that she was upstaged to Stage IV. She had a thoracic wedge resection of the metastasis and began receiving what Tony described as a "five-drug cocktail" of chemotherapeutic agents, as well as an aromatase inhibitor. Despite the grave prognosis and recent major surgery, Sherrie Antoszewski participated in the 3-Day event with Tony and the other members of their training group. In all, there were 103 members on their team—the largest team at the Michigan walk that year.

As mentioned, Sherrie achieved remission; however, her twin sister was not as fortunate. Dawn was diagnosed with brain metastases a few months before Tony participated in the 2004 Breast Cancer 3-Day event. Pinned to Tony's back was a laminated copy of a newspaper article about his wife and sister-in-law. The article described a fundraiser that had taken place a few weeks before, to raise money for Dawn's treatment. "They're very close, Sherrie and Dawn. Dawn's very free spirited. I joke with her. I've always called her an airhead. So now, it's metastasized to the brain, and I go up to her and say, 'You're still an airhead, but you're my favorite airhead.'" Tony paused to compose himself. "We're not giving up. If Dawn makes it two years … what can happen in the next two years in the medical field? Could be something. If they wouldn't have found it, she wouldn't have made it six months."

Although Tony Antoszewski was an only child, he would have made a terrific big brother, as shown by the tenderness he expressed toward his sister-in-law and by how supportive he was toward one of his and Sherrie's 2002 teammates, Kim Hochstettler, 26, who was also walking in 2004. From their interactions, it was clear that Kim saw Tony as a trusted older brother.

Kim's mother died of breast cancer in 1999, just a few months before Kim and her husband's son was born. Kim viewed the 2002 3-Day event as a critical step in coming to terms with her mother's death and an important way to honor her memory; however, Kim's husband declined to participate in the 3-Day and even trivialized the emotional significance of her participation. Kim said, "He asked me, 'Do you want me to bring Evan down for Closing Ceremonies?'—Evan is our son—and I said, 'Do you really have to ask me that?' I just looked at him and said, 'You *know* what this means to me. You *know* why I'm doing this. *Do you have to ask me that?*'" Kim's voice shook as she said the last sentence.

"Over the course of the [2002] walk, I decided I needed to do something about it. The walk was in June and I filed for divorce on November 1. It took me a while to get up the guts to go down to the courthouse, but I filed, and he moved out. The divorce was final in July."

Kim became friends with Tony and Sherrie Antoszewski during training walks for the 2002 Michigan 3-Day. They have remained friends since then and their children play together. In fact, her friendships with the Antoszewskis and an old high-school friend were Kim's support system during her divorce. About her father, Kim said, "He's been an alcoholic his whole life and got worse when my mother passed away." Kim has a brother, but he, too, had recently gone through a divorce and was unable to provide much emotional support to Kim.

As Kim related the details of her mother's protracted illness and eventual death from breast cancer, Tony listened sympathetically and patted Kim on the shoulder when she intermittently cried. Despite the disappointment of her divorce and the profound sadness about her mother's death, Kim expressed optimism about the future. Like an encouraging older brother, Tony said, "Kim, you're in a completely different place than you were before. You're doing so good."

When Tony wrote down his contact information, I looked at the address on Woodward Avenue and a little jingle sounded in my head. "Woodward. *Woodward.* Why does that sound so familiar to me?" I asked.

Tony said, "Maybe the Woodward Dream Cruise?"

"Of course," I said. "I read about it in the newspaper."

An article by Nick Bunkley in the August 18, 2004, issue of *The Detroit News*, entitled "Woodward Dream Cruise," had reported: "Saturday, August 21 is the 10th anniversary of Motown's homage to the car culture of the '50s and '60s. About 40,000 street rods, muscle cars and customized vehicles will flood Woodward from Eight Mile to Pontiac for Saturday's cruise. The world's largest one-day auto event, the Dream Cruise, is expected to draw more than 1 million fans along the 16-mile route that became a legendary cruising strip in the 1950s ..."

One million fans. That number was staggering, incomprehensible, but so are the sheer numbers of women who will be diagnosed with breast cancer. Let's say that roughly half the fans lining Woodward Avenue are women. That would be 500,000. Given that a woman has a one in seven chance of developing breast cancer during her lifetime, this means that approximately 70,000 of those women have either had breast cancer or will develop breast cancer during her lifetime—some of those breast cancers will occur in men, too. Nearly three times that many—200,000—will be diagnosed with breast cancer every year in the United States.

While those women and men, and their families and friends, watched the cars, about 1,650 walkers were walking Day 2 of the Michigan 3-Day. Our route took us through Plymouth, Northville, and Livonia. Pit Stop 3 at 15.5 miles was at the Henry Ford Medical Center of Livonia. According to the Henry Ford Health System Web site (www.henryford.com), there are four Josephine Ford Cancer Centers in their system, which are "comprehensive cancer centers located about 20 minutes from any patient in southeast Michigan." Henry Ford Medical Center at Livonia—our Pit Stop 3—was one of the 11 accredited mammography centers that serve the Josephine Ford Cancer Centers, which is "the largest mammography provider in Michigan." Those centers "serve over 60,000 women annually." That's still 10,000 shy of the 70,000 present and future breast cancer patients among the fans of the Woodward Dream Cruise.

One of the first people that I met during the Michigan 3-Day was breast cancer survivor Sally Krause. She and her walking buddy, Roberta, invited me to join them at their table during breakfast at the host hotel on Day 1. Host hotels invariably provided 3-Day participants with breakfast snacks and beverages before we boarded the shuttle buses at 5 AM to go to Opening Ceremonies. They either opened their continental breakfast bars early (4:30 AM) or set up beverage- and snack-laden tables in the lobbies.

I saw Sally and Roberta again during the second day, and we walked together awhile. We talked about our grown children, and Sally bragged (in a very civilized way, of course) about her grandchildren. Before we parted, she asked if it would be okay if we walked together at Closing Ceremonies. I said, "Absolutely."

As I had done before Closing Ceremonies in New York and Washington, D.C., I found a relatively quiet place for a short nap, away from the crowds, as I waited for the ceremony to begin. When I awoke, the participants were already lining up for the final walk. I gathered up my fanny pack and pink shirt, and scrambled to join the flock of pinkies. At first, I didn't see Sally and wondered if she had given up on me and found someone else to walk beside.

I put on my pink shirt and side-stepped along the edge of the survivor group, counting the rows: 14 rows, six walkers in each. Sally spotted me and tugged me by the arm to the back of the group. She was carrying a small bouquet of orange roses that one of her grandchildren had brought for her. She told me that her entire family was there to greet her: her husband, two sons, two daughters-in-law, and three grandchildren, the youngest of which was in a stroller. As we waited to begin the victory walk, she cell-phoned her family to let them know that she was in the last row on the right.

As we slowly approached the stage, Sally pointed out her family. "The young woman in the yellow tank top—that's my daughter-in-law. The man behind her waving is my son." A blonde-haired little girl, about five years old, scampered out from the cheering crowd, squeezed Sally around her hips, and ran back. As we approached her cheering family, her tall, trim, gray-haired husband stepped from the crowd and, without a word, pulled her toward him. Cradling her head in his hands, he gave her a long, hungry kiss, worthy of a returning soldier. He back-stepped into the crowd, smiling, gazing at her with an expression of unrestrained love and pride. Sally's sons and daughters-in-law were clapping and cheering, but her husband stood with his hands at his sides, continuing to gaze at her, tears coming to his eyes.

If people saw me crying, they probably thought it had to do with the power of Closing Ceremonies, but that wasn't it. By any yardstick, I was having the biggest adventure of my life, traveling all over the country to participate in 3-Day events. Adventure or not, it didn't prevent me from getting homesick. I missed my mom and my little sisters; my children, Jessica and Andrew; and my friends, René, Beth, Cathy, and Linda. I missed my pets and my backyard and my creaky old house. I missed cooking supper and wearing perfume and building my rock wall. Most of all, though, I missed Tom, my sweet, gentle fiancé. I missed him every day that I was gone; however, it wasn't until I saw Sally Krause's husband kiss her that I began to wonder if the project justified being away from him.

I was seriously considering shelving the whole damn-fool project until my friends Bob and Barbara Jo Kirshbaum took me out to dinner that evening at Ruth's Chris Steak House to celebrate my birthday. Over coffee and crème broulee, they delivered a gentle, much-needed pep talk. As we parted, I said, "See y'all in Chicago."

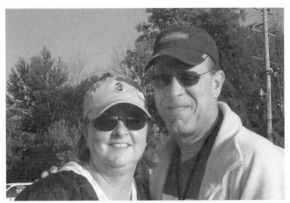

Gale and Tim Colston

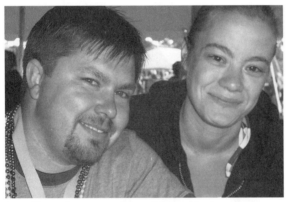

Tony Antoszewski and Kim Hochstettler

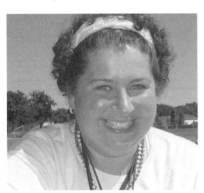

Kim Clexton

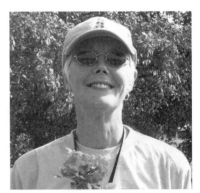

Sally Krause

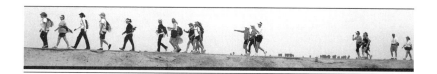

Chapter 5

Chicago
August 27, August 28, and August 29, 2004

Thursday, August 26, 2004, was Day 0 for the Chicago 3-Day. It was also the day that the world's most famous women's sports team stood on the gold medal platform at the 2004 Olympic Games in Athens, Greece. With pluck and luck, the American women's soccer team beat the favored Brazilian team in the 22nd minute of overtime. Among those wearing gold medals and laurels were Mia Hamm, Kristine Lilly, Julie Foudy, Brandi Chastain, and Joy Fawcett—five women's soccer pioneers. These five women had been on the team that won soccer's first Women's World Cup in 1991 in China and on the team that won the first Olympic gold medal in 1996 in Athens, Georgia.

Some of the 91ers—as Mia Hamm and the other veterans were called by their younger teammates—were playing their final international game at the 2004 Olympics. Taking home the gold medal would be a crowning glory for their careers, but going into the Olympics was far from inevitable. The team had not won a major championship since the 1999 World Cup, when Brandi Chastain left-footed a penalty kick and whipped off her t-shirt at the Rose Bowl. An estimated 40 million Americans watched the game on television. According to an article posted by Grant Wahl on July 23, 1999, on the CNN/Sports Illustrated Web site (SI.com), "… the Cup final was the most watched soccer match in the history of network television, and the turnout of 90,185 at the Rose Bowl was the largest ever at a women's sporting event."

My husband, Andy, and I were among those 40 million Americans watching our women's soccer team win the World Cup on July 10, 1999. When Brandi Chastain nailed her penalty kick, I jumped up from where I was sitting on the edge of Andy's bed and sprinted in place, arms pumping. I whooped, "Yes!" and wept. I could not have been more pleased had my own daughter been on the team. In a way, I felt like they *were* my daughters. After all, it had been *my* generation of women— those of us who had come of age in the wake of Betty Friedan's book,

The Feminine Mystique—who bludgeoned pathways through what was called "a glass ceiling," but which was, in truth, more like a labyrinth of tricky mirrors.

As our women's soccer team hugged and jumped for joy, ponytails bouncing, Andy clapped in slow motion and smiled. By that point he weighed less than a hundred pounds, took his meals in bed, and needed assistance going to the bathroom. I took showers with him, steadying him as I washed him from head to toe, while he leaned against the tile wall. Near the end, most of our conversations were my questions about his comfort and his short responses: "Are you cool/warm enough?" "Would you like some more ice chips/apple juice/Sprite?" "How about a nice foot rub/back rub/head rub?"

Our days ebbed and flowed between his doses of Roxanol®—a rapid-acting morphine sulfate that he took by mouth every four hours. I needed his morphine as much as he did. As his blood level ebbed, he would begin to squint his eyes. This was the first subtle indication that his pain was returning. I became restless and remained so until he allowed me to put the bitter medicine onto the back of his tongue with an eyedropper. As he relaxed, so did I. It is not histrionic to say that, had it been neces-sary, I would have sold my soul to get morphine for Andy.

During Andy's last few months, and especially the last few weeks, we watched a lot of television together. That's how I came to see Mia Hamm, Brianna Scurry, and the others win the World Cup. The day they won (July 10, 1999) was also Andy and my 23rd wedding anniver-sary. I told him that we could call their victory our anniversary celebra-tion. He grinned and said, "Well, it's cheaper than taking you out to Ruth's Chris."

On August 6, 1999, the day before he died, Andy became increas-ingly confused and unresponsive. Although I didn't know it until later, he was bleeding into a brain metastasis. That afternoon he had a grand mal seizure. Drifting peacefully to his death at home was one thing, but hav-ing seizures with our children nearby was quite another.

I called an ambulance. I then called a long-time family friend and neighbor, Linda Ybarra, and asked her to stay with our children. As we waited long minutes for the ambulance to arrive, our children were cry-ing and frantic. I tried to soothe them and comfort Andy, hoping that he wouldn't have another seizure before help arrived. Andy was stuttering badly but was still trying to talk. As he was being lifted onto the transport gurney, he was saying our children's names and repeating, "I love you."

Sobbing and choking on their words, they were both saying, "Daddy, I love you. Daddy, I love you."

In the ambulance, on the way to the hospital with Andy, I wasn't praying. I also didn't pray during his brief, final hospitalization. Instead, I was cursing God, and I would continue to curse God for a long time. During the year and a half that Andy was sick, I had been intermittently angry; however, after he died a horrible death, I seethed inside almost every waking moment. Impatient? Inexcusably so.

My anger couldn't protect me from my dreams, though. I frequently woke up in the darkness and cried. Then, I would get up the next morning and go to work, puffy-eyed but smiling, and put on a good show—at least most of the time. Unfortunately, my anger would sometimes erupt and flatten an unsuspecting (and, for the most part, undeserving) target. Friends and genuinely kind, caring acquaintances were not spared from my appalling behavior.

Not until I walked beside Debby Padzensky at the Chicago 3-Day did I realize that my anger and refusal to accept comfort were not simply the residue from a lifetime of stubborn independence, but rather indications of a lack of humanness. When Debby was diagnosed with breast cancer at age 33, she readily accepted help from many sources, including the group of friends who were walking on her team at the 3-Day. Debby was willing to receive help because, with every molecule in her body, she is willing to give help. For her, to be human is to be able to give *and to receive* help from others.

Debby is a social worker and job-shares with another social worker at an elementary school attended by children from disadvantaged families. She works primarily with students who are causing problems in class—"loving the children that other people don't love." She described her job this way: "I take care of other people, their feelings, and their behaviors; their problems and conflicts … I'm a therapist. I help people deal with their feelings and communicate. My way is to talk it out. Talk, talk, talk. People talk, use their words, bring things to the surface."

In short, she considers vigorous communication indispensable for solving problems. Her emphasis on being able to communicate led her to interview four medical oncologists before beginning treatment with Dr. Jacob Bitran, whom she referred to as "Dr. B." The medical training and professional reputations of all four medical oncologists whom she interviewed were exemplary; however, Dr. Bitran's skills at communicating and listening were the deciding factors for Debby.

She explained, "I'm not just someone who says 'okay' when someone says go to this person for treatment. I do my research. I have to go to people whom I'm really comfortable with. They can be brilliant doctors, but if they have a poor bedside manner, and I can't ask questions or I'm intimidated or feel like they're rushing things, I can't go to them."

Her insistence on a communicative doctor proved wise, since her breast disease was complicated and she needed aggressive treatment. First of all, she had two separate invasive carcinomas in her breast. Secondly, her tumors overexpressed *HER-2/neu*. Finally, like her father, who had been diagnosed with breast cancer two years before Debby was diagnosed, she was positive for *BRCA2*. More so, perhaps, than some breast cancer patients, she needed a medical oncologist who could help her consider the options and weigh the possible benefits of adjuvant therapies. To borrow her phrase, she needed to "talk, talk, talk" in order to make informed decisions.

Debby's father was 64 years old and a highly successful business-man when he found a lump in his chest. His internist referred him to a surgeon who did a biopsy. To everyone's surprise, including Debby's, the lump turned out to be breast cancer. "It wasn't something we were expecting. Prostate cancer, maybe, or a heart attack, but not *breast* can-cer ... I was 30 at the time and just had my first son. It was frightening to hear that my father had cancer, but breast cancer didn't seem too worri-some in a man. If it had been my mom who had been diagnosed with breast cancer, it would have hit me in a different way. Honestly, it was scary, but I didn't really worry. I thought, It's never going to get to my dad, because he's strong, he's physically strong. He wasn't very tall, but he was very stocky. He had these big hands from playing handball for a gazillion years. It didn't seem like anything that would ever take his life or get to him ... Breast cancer in my dad? It just didn't make sense. So our attitude was that we'll take care of business and move on."

For Debby's father, "taking care of business" began with a mastec-tomy and axillary node dissection. Three of his axillary lymph nodes were positive for metastatic carcinoma. Debby's father received four rounds of combination chemotherapy at three-week intervals, six weeks of radiation treatment, followed by tamoxifen. In short, his treatment for breast cancer was no different than it would have been for a woman with the same disease stage; however, her father's reaction to his diagnosis and treatment was definitely gender-specific. "His hairy chest covered the lack of a nipple so you wouldn't have noticed unless you were really focusing. It wasn't emotionally difficult for him either. My father's sense of himself, besides being proud of his wife and his daughters, was his business and working. That he couldn't work was the disruptive part for him."

Debby is the youngest of three daughters and, because of their father's diagnosis, early screening mammograms were recommended. When her older sisters were scheduling their mammograms, Debby was pregnant with her second child and elected to wait until after she deliv-ered to have a mammogram. "I had my baby. A year later, I was nursing, and I stopped nursing in June 1999. In September, I went to the doctor for an appointment and asked, 'When should I have a mammogram? My dad had breast cancer, and I'm 33.' She said, 'Wait until you're 35, unless you're going to have another child, then have the mammogram beforehand.' Having another child would have been my plan.

"The doctor said, 'Lie down,' and she did a breast exam. She could feel the lumps. They were there. I just didn't ..." Debby's voice trailed off, she shook her head, then paused before speaking again. "Your breasts get lumpy from nursing. While I was nursing my second child, I just wasn't in touch with my body. They were there."

Debby, her husband, and their two young sons were in the process of moving from Chicago to the suburb of Deerfield when the breast masses were discovered. "We had to live with my in-laws for a few weeks while we waited for our house. It was during that time that I had to wait. Initially I went to Northwestern, which is a nationally known facility, but they're so busy at the Breast Center there that I had to wait a week or so to get a mammogram. They saw something [on the first mammogram], so they called me back. My husband was in the waiting room and we were trying to be positive.

"I was waiting in the room with all these women who were older than I was. It was scary because I didn't think I should be in this group. I went back for the repeat mammogram and said, 'Now, why are we doing this?' and they said, 'Well, sometimes we don't get a clear view.' I went back out to the waiting room again and was beginning to get nervous. Then they came and said, 'We're going to have to do an ultrasound to get a better picture.'

"I walked out into the hall with my husband and started crying. I said, 'They want to take an ultrasound, and they're not telling me that anything's wrong. Why would they want to do this if something weren't wrong?'

"The radiologist didn't tell me it was cancer until after they had done the biopsy, but they knew. For example, the nurse who walked out with me said, 'I just recovered from ovarian cancer and things will be okay.' She was indirectly telling me. She wanted to tell me that I was going to be okay because they knew."

It was another week and a half before the biopsies of the suspicious masses were done—first, fine-needle aspiration biopsies; later, core biopsies. Debby said, "Those 10 days were probably the worst days of the whole experience. I lost the most weight then. I functioned well—nobody would know—but I was anxious and worried. I kept thinking, Well, what if it is? What if it isn't?" Debby leaned her head first to one side, then the other, as she recalled her bewilderment. "Why would they say this? It probably means this. If they said this, maybe it's not. Just back and forth and back and forth. I was just *crazy*.

"It was helpful during this time to go to work because I thought, Well, my problems are small in comparison to what these people are going through, but at this point, I was getting a little worried because cancer is *not* such a small problem. Looking back, I could have gone anywhere and had these tests done so much more quickly. There was no reason for me to wait but I didn't know."

Debby pointed toward the five women walking ahead of us who were on her 3-Day team, Ron's Ribbons. (Debby's father was named Ron. Throughout the Chicago 3-Day event, she wore a photograph of him pinned to her back.) "That's my group up there. I've known three of them since I was 10 years old. Breast cancer isn't the kind of thing women our age struggle with. I was the first one in our group, so I just *didn't know.*

"I had to have a couple of different types of biopsy. The next day, I missed work. That day I was waiting, waiting, waiting for the call. Finally, at 6 o'clock, the radiologist called and said, 'We got the results back, and I'm really sorry but you have cancer.'

Debby snapped her head back, like she'd been punched. "After I hung up the phone I thought, So what do I *do* with this information? One of my best girlfriends is married to an oncologist. He's a love. He worked out of M.D. Anderson, then Northwestern, and now he's at the group by us. They came over to our house. I was lucky that I had that resource ... He is a mensch. He came by and talked to me. He answered questions like, 'Will I be needing chemo?' 'Will I be needing a mastectomy?' Things like that."

Like her previously described approach to choosing an oncologist, Debby set about interviewing surgeons. "I needed to have a mastectomy. I knew that, at some point down the road, I would need to do the other side, but I thought I would start with one. Although some people choose to do both sides at once, I just didn't want to do that. I needed to take care of my kids. A bilateral mastectomy would have prolonged my recovery, so I just did one side. I had to decide if I wanted to do recontruction immediately, so I kept going back and forth and back and forth, talking to people, searching the Internet, reading. It was just crazy. I couldn't decide. Okay, I finally thought, I need to make a decision. I knew that a TRAM [transverse rectus abdominis myocutaneous flap reconstruction] would take longer to recover, so I decided to have a tissue expander put in."

While recovering from surgery she researched treatment protocols and interviewed medical oncologists. "I had nine positive nodes. I'm estrogen-receptor (ER) positive and I'm young. It's more aggressive in younger women. I was *HER-2* [*HER-2/neu*] positive and that's often a more aggressive kind. The standard protocol was A/C [Adriamycin® and Cytoxan®] every three weeks and then, for me, they would have added Taxol® [paclitaxel] every two weeks. I also knew that I was a candidate for Herceptin® [trastuzumab]. I did my research about that, and some said maybe; others said maybe not. It has been FDA-approved for women in Stage IV, but we didn't know for sure. There was a study going on.

"Then I went to see Dr. B. from the University of Chicago. [Dr. Jacob Bitran now practices at Lutheran General Cancer Care Center in Park Ridge, Illinois.] His CV is pretty impressive and he's just a nice man. He wanted to do something more aggressive. He said, 'Let's put you in the 10-plus range for lymph node involvement.' I said, 'Great. What do we do?'"

Instead of receiving standard-dose combination chemotherapy, which is every three weeks, Dr. Bitran recommended dose-dense treatment, which means that the interval between treatments is shortened to two weeks. Debby received an equivalent dose of chemotherapy but within a shorter period of time—every two weeks instead of every three weeks. Patients, like Debby, who receive chemotherapy at an increased frequency, require bone marrow growth factors such as filgrastim (Neupogen®) and pegfilgrastim (Neulasta®) to avoid life-threatening infections from drops in white blood cell counts.

Dr. Bitran explained that the Adriamycin® was at a high dose, just shy of the dose used for patients who are undergoing stem cell transplant. Debby said, "At that time [1999], the studies showed that the stem cell transplants weren't as effective or as promising as they thought they'd be. It's not worth it to go through all that. The one study comparing stem cell transplant with this dose-dense treatment favored dose-dense. I told him that I was really scared to do stem cell. Sure, I wanted to live, and if he had told me that I needed to do that, then I would have done it, but he said, 'Honestly, Debby, if you were my sister, I would do dose-dense treatment, and I can do that for you here.' I said, 'Great.'"

The results of what was considered by many to be a landmark study of dose-dense treatment were not reported until 2003 in an article in the *Journal of Clinical Oncology*. Dr. Marc L. Citron and other researchers showed that dose-dense treatment improved both the overall and the disease-free survival. Still, Dr. Bitran recommended this approach to Debby in 1999.

"My friend's husband, who is the medical oncologist, had shown me the literature that came out of the San Antonio Breast Cancer Symposium last year [2003] indicating that dose-dense is the way to go. Dr. B. didn't know for sure but said he had a good feeling about it. I never wound up in the hospital but I had the usual symptoms throughout chemotherapy. I can't imagine how people do two drugs together even though they have three weeks in between. With the Adriamycin®, I had a dry mouth and a metallic taste. I have a very weak stomach to begin with, so my main issue was finding things that weren't going to upset my gastrointestinal system.

"With the Taxol®, I had really bad headaches that Tylenol® couldn't touch." Debby clenched her fists and tapped them lightly together a couple of times. "After the second treatment, I told them about the headaches and they said, 'Why didn't you call us the first time?' They prescribed prednisone and I was like *woo-hoo*." She laughed and said, "I'm not a great house cleaner but I was mopping the floors! I felt better than I had in a lo-o-o-ng time.

"With Cytoxan®, I'd throw up within an hour, literally, before I walked out the door. After I came home, I'd be wiped out for about a day and then I'd be fine. Not *fine*, but pretty fine.

"I was very, very fortunate because of my support network. There was my husband, Ron, who is just the most amazing man. He is such a hands-on father. Then there were my two sisters who live five minutes from me, east; my mother-in-law who lives five minutes from me, west; my mother who lives 20 minutes away; and my grandmother—my nana. I would not have gotten through this without their love and support. My family was just amazing—totally, totally amazing. And these guys," motioning toward her teammates, "were great. They organized meals. I had a cleaning lady every other week but they filled in the week that I didn't have one ... Do you remember when your kids were little, that bad time of the day, late in the afternoon when they're cranky but it's not yet time for bed? You really have to struggle to keep them occupied."

I nodded and said, "Oh, yeah. We used to call it 'whiney hour.'"

Pointing toward her teammates, she said, "They would come and stay with me to conserve my energy. Even though I would say, 'I can do it,' they would say, 'We're coming.' I was on such a high during my treatment. Afterwards I had a big barbecue in my backyard to thank everyone who helped."

Debby started chemotherapy in early December 1999 and finished at the end of March of the following year. Following chemotherapy she received radiation treatment through June, after which she received Herceptin® for six months (until November 2000). After her first dose of chemotherapy she stopped menstruating and, despite delaying the initiation of tamoxifen treatment in hopes that she would begin cycling again, she never menstruated after that. "I didn't start on tamoxifen right away because I wanted to have more children. That was just so tough emotionally. I couldn't believe that that choice was taken away from me. I went into menopause right after the first treatment and never got it back. Dr. B. didn't seem to think there was any rush that I start on tamoxifen so I waited six months. In the interim, I was going to Northwestern on the ovarian cancer study with Dr. David Fishman."

The study to which Debby was referring is the National Ovarian Cancer Early Detection Program at Northwestern University. David A. Fishman, M.D., directs the program, which is a collaborative effort between the National Cancer Institute, Northwestern University, and the Robert H. Lurie Comprehensive Cancer Center of Northwestern. In contrast to overall breast cancer survival statistics, which have dramatically improved because of earlier detection, a way to detect ovarian cancer at an early, treatable stage has remained elusive. Dr. Fishman and other researchers are looking for a method to screen all women by studying those who may be at greater risk. Those who are eligible for the study include women who have had breast, colon, or urinary tract cancer; women with a mother, sister, or daughter with ovarian cancer; women with multiple family members with either breast and/or ovarian cancer; women who have a *BRCA1* or *BRCA2* gene mutation or whose close relative has one of the gene mutations; and women who have used fertility drugs for more than a year.

Obviously Debby was a candidate from several standpoints. She was a breast cancer survivor, she had multiple family members with breast cancer (not only her dad, but also a great-aunt and her dad's cousin), and she and her dad were carriers of the *BRCA2* gene mutation. People with *BRCA* gene mutations have an inherited predisposition for developing cancer. Women with *BRCA* gene mutations have a lifetime risk of breast cancer that approaches 85% compared to a 13% risk for women without these gene mutations. They also have a sobering increase in the incidence of ovarian cancer.

Shortly after Debby was diagnosed with breast cancer, her father developed a chronic cough. "His internist, from what I can remember, was trying cough medicine and Tylenol® with codeine. I thought that, once you've had cancer, you always think about that first and consult your oncologist. Anyway, he did have tumor markers done, and they were normal in October. Three months later, when my parents returned home from a trip to Mexico, my mother took him right to the hospital because he was coughing so much. They took their time figuring things out before they told us, but I knew from being in my groups how it happened. I'm too cancer-wise so I wasn't surprised." Debby shook her head and paused before continuing.

"When they did the tumor markers three months later, the level had skyrocketed. The tumor was there before but hadn't shown up with the tumor markers. He didn't have the follow-up like I had with Dr. B. For two years I had a CAT [computerized axial tomography] scan and a bone scan every six months, then yearly after that for five years. My dad didn't have any of that done. I think he had a chest x-ray at some point, but if he would have had those kinds of tests, they would have seen it … I was in the middle of taking Taxol® [when my father was diagnosed with metastatic disease] and he was immediately put on Taxol®. We were on it together but with different doctors. We sort of made jokes about it. He'd call me and say, 'I have a really bad headache. Do you get this?' and I'd say, 'No, sorry, Dad. I guess I'm healthier than you.'" Debby smiled slowly but cleared her throat before continuing.

"Later, it was in his brain; it was in his bones; it was in his lungs. He had the gamma knife surgery on his brain twice. There were 17 lesions in his brain. He went off the tamoxifen. That's the other thing. I wound up taking his tamoxifen when he went off it. I never really felt good about taking his rejects because they hadn't worked for him. It wound up causing tumors on my liver. They've been closely watching those for two and a half years, and I do believe they are benign now. They test them every six months, and they haven't changed. The oncologist has always believed they were benign."

She turned her head to look directly at me. I sensed that she wanted me to offer my medical opinion about the significance of her liver masses but, instead, I said, "It sounds like they're following you very closely." Debby was medically very sophisticated. She no doubt understood my reluctance to trivialize the possible gravity of liver masses in a young woman who had presented with locally advanced disease. I think my concern mirrored hers. She nodded and pressed her lips together before continuing.

"All of 2000, my dad was sick. The doctors wouldn't tell him that he had recurrent cancer, but that was what was going on and I knew it … Then his kidneys began to fail. In December 2000, he started dialysis, and in January, he died. We were literally standing there when he took his last breath—my sisters and my mother and I … He was in a coma, but he woke up and turned and looked—not at my sisters or me—but right at my mom for 30 seconds. Then he took his last breath and he was gone … I still can't explain that." Debby nodded her head slowly, her eyes shining. She swallowed before adding, her voice husky, "It was the most beautiful way to die."

Throughout much of her father's final year, Debby was undergoing adjuvant therapy. She was also mothering two young boys and working at the elementary school. Although she had support from her family and friends, she joined a cancer patient support group for women at the Cancer Wellness Center/Barbara Kassel Brotman House in Northbrook, Illinois.

"I went to the support group for a year and a half … I walked in and there were about 10 people, the majority of whom were under 40. Most of us were breast cancer [patients] but there were other cancers, too. It took me a few times [to feel comfortable] because there were people in there who were dying … By talking with some of these women, I was able to stare death in the face. I was 33 years old and had never lost anyone in my whole life. It wasn't something that I was comfortable with. We don't have wakes. In the Jewish religion, we don't view the bodies often. It's not something we're comfortable with, but the women in that group taught me about facing death with such dignity.

"They helped me when my father had cancer again. I could talk to these people about my dad because they were not as emotionally involved as, say, my mother and sisters. My family was focused on being optimistic about Dad's prognosis, so I was reluctant to say, 'I think Dad is getting cancer again.' I didn't want to worry my mother and sisters until I knew what was happening, but I could tell the people in my group that I knew my dad was going to die.

"From the group, I learned that you do whatever it takes. With this disease there's no right or wrong way. There are right and wrong things to *do* in life, but no right or wrong way to handle cancer." (Debby, of course, had just stated—very eloquently—one of the intended messages of this book.)

"The Cancer Wellness Center is perfect for me. It's funded through donations and grants. In October, they have an annual benefit with a lot of corporate sponsorship. It's a beautiful facility with gorgeous support group rooms. There's a round tai chi room that overlooks a pond. There's a beautiful library, a kitchen, and a huge meeting room. Everything's free, so I even get massages there. I've tried healing touch. I've done visualization imaging classes. Plus, they have tons of seminars taught by professionals, so that I can get CEUs [Continuing Education Units] for my license.

"About six months ago, I attended a conference for CEUs called Couples in Cancer. There were people from the University of Chicago specializing in sexuality and intimacy and couples coping. They pointed out that when life is going along fine, couples can manage, but when there's a crisis and their ways of coping aren't always working, they have to find new ways. A lot of people don't have extra tools to deal with that … The seminar covered some of the same territory that Ron and I dealt with when I was going through treatment. For instance, he's in information technology and he's very task oriented. He enters into task mode. I need to talk, talk, talk, and I can get overwhelmed with emotion.

"Luckily, he was really good at being able to kick into task mode to get through things. When it was all over, though, I needed something else … With everybody else I'm very upbeat and positive and cheerful—a poster child. With him, I needed to be able to talk … There were some tough times—times that tested our marriage—but he was amazing. Looking back, I think that, at times, my expectations were unrealistic. On one hand, I wanted him to be strong, but then, on the other hand, I wanted him to show me that he was scared, too.

"The year of treatment was hellish. You're on autopilot all those months and then you finish and you're like, 'Whoa, *what the hell*? What the hell's happening? Omigod, what was *that*?' You take it in and then you wonder how you're going to go on. You're trying to find a balance between what happened and the new perspective that you didn't ask for … Then you end up waiting for the next appointment.

"After treatment finished, I had been going in monthly. Then I was on to my three-month plan. That was hard. Every year, it's gotten easier but it's always in the back of my mind—that little voice that says my reality is that it could still be there. When I was going in every six months for CAT scans and bone scans, I would always think, This could be the day that changes my whole life forever if I find out there's a malignancy there. My whole life would change. My husband didn't really know how to help at those times. He couldn't possibly read my mind and know what I wanted him to say.

"My support group said, 'Debby, you need to tell him what you need. You've got to *constantly* be telling him what you need.'

"I said, 'I feel like he should know. That just seems obvious to me.'

"Then one of them said, 'It's *not* obvious. He's *not* the one with cancer. No one can really know what it's like in your skin.'

"So I got better at learning to ask and not just expecting him to know what I needed. I've also gotten better about not getting upset. I'm on the Outreach Committee at the Cancer Wellness Center so I know a lot of people who have breast cancer. I'm always at a higher risk than everyone I know, and I would sometimes think, How am I going to make it? It was almost considered normal for most of them to survive, so they would tell me, 'Oh, you're going to be fine. You're doing fine.'

"Those people don't really understand how advanced my cancer was by the time it was found. They don't really understand my reality ... I even did the same thing to my dad a time or two. I also realized that I was going to the support group and saying the same things to the people there that I didn't like said to me—things like, 'Oh, you'll be fine.' For instance, when my dad was dying and in a coma, a friend came to the hospital and found me in the hall sobbing. I said, 'That is going to happen to me,' and she said, 'No, it won't, Debby,' and I said, 'Yeah, it could. This could be a reality.'

"She said, 'I know, Debby, but you need to focus on the good stuff and the positives.' I told her, 'I *do* focus on the positives, but there are times when the bad stuff seeps in.'

"It gets bad around anniversaries and appointments ... I definitely have days when I'm angry that it happened. I'm angry that this is my reality. That's why I make this walk. It rejuvenates me. It reminds me how many people are diagnosed; how many people are dying; how many people are having the kind of life that I had for those few years; how many people might not have the kind of support that I had.

"Like I said in my thank-you note for my first 3-Day walk, I learned a life lesson at 33 years old that some people never learn. In a way, I feel sorry for those people who will never have that kind of enrichment ... Truly, as long as I continue to survive this, it will continue to enrich my life. I've seen my friends change. It shook everybody up. It was a wake-up call ... Last night at camp, we had a ton of people. Numerous friends have had babies, or this or that, and couldn't walk, but they came to visit us at camp. We had a big slumber party up in our classroom. All of our kids were there and our friends. It's really touched their lives in a very positive way—to really experience what it is to do good for other people, to go beyond yourself and your life, and to really care about a cause."

When Debby said "up in our classroom," she was referring to one of the classrooms at Old Orchard Junior High School in Skokie. We were supposed to camp on the school grounds at the end of Day 2; however, it was raining. Although we ate dinner and breakfast in the big dining tent and showered in the semi-trucks, walkers and crew "camped out" in the classrooms and hallways of Old Orchard Junior High School.

One reason that "a ton of people" came to visit Debby is that she and some of her teammates grew up in Skokie.

The next day the route wound through Skokie before entering Chicago. I walked with Debby and her teammates, as these "Skokie girls," as some of the other walkers had dubbed them, traded childhood memories. It was a beautiful day for being nostalgic. Unlike Days 1 and 2, Day 3 was blue-skied and breezy—a perfect day to fly kites, buy ice cream from a bell-ringing vendor, and walk the final miles along Lake Michigan to Lincoln Park.

In fact, until Day 3 of the Chicago event, the weather played cat-and-mouse with us. On Day 1, when we arrived at Tremper High School in Kenosha, Wisconsin, for Opening Ceremonies, an overnight storm had tipped—and, in some cases, knocked over—the porta-potties. To our relief, two porta-potty service people arrived at 6 AM. Mighty Mouse himself couldn't have worked any faster to correct the problem. The lines of waiting (and squirming) women cheered and applauded their super-efforts.

This is as good a time as any to talk "porta-potty." Prior to the 3-Day, the utterance of this phrase evoked dread. One of the stronger memories involved a big soccer tournament on a blazing South Texas day. Stepping into and closing the door of that porta-potty couldn't have been much worse than stepping into the very fires of hell. In addition to the ungodly heat were the sounds of buzzing flies, the stickiness of the floor, the smell of ...

Suffice it to say that my many, many pleasant trips to porta-potties at 3-Day events across the country have, if not completely wiped away the soccer tournament memory, certainly sanitized my limbic brain response to the phrase.

At the risk of seeming a little peculiar (notice that I didn't say "anal retentive"), I figured out that my walnut-sized bladder and I made about 400 visits to porta-potties during the 2004 3-Day events. In other words, I sit (or, with some frequency, sat) in the position to judge the insides of these modern-day outhouses. Here's my verdict: With very rare, and always excusable (or passing), exceptions, the porta-potties were clean, fresh smelling, and well supplied with toilet paper. Some Pit Stop crews even taped jokes or inspirational sayings, trivia questions, and photos of hunky guys on the inside of the doors.

There's no graceful way to move from porta-potties to the next section other than to say that I recognized Mark Bornstein in the porta-potty line at the first Pit Stop after Opening Ceremonies on Day 1. Mark had read the Circle of Spirit part at the Chicago 3-Day Opening Ceremonies and his wife, Tammi, was one of the women in the Survivors' Circle. It was a departure from the usual for anyone but Nancy Mercurio, national spokesperson for the Breast Cancer 3-Day, to read the Survivors' Circle part of Opening Ceremonies.

There was another departure from the usual Opening Ceremonies at Chicago. At most of the 3-Day events Pat (Patrice) Tosi, chief operating officer and executive vice president of the Susan G. Komen Foundation, was onstage at Opening and Closing Ceremonies. At most Opening Ceremonies, Ms. Tosi reported the number of participants and the amount of money raised. She also described how the Susan G. Komen Foundation came into being as "a promise between two sisters"; however, at the Chicago 3-Day, Susan Braun, who was then president and chief executive officer of the Komen Foundation, was that organization's representative. Ms. Braun told us that 1,570 walkers and 255 volunteer crew members were participating and congratulated us on raising $4.3 million. She also introduced Mark for the Circle of Spirit reading.

Tammi and Mark Bornstein have been married for 14 years. Even before you hear their tender verbal exchanges and their shared laughter at a funny story, their body language and mannerisms indicate that they have a solid marriage. (Granted, mine is not a professional opinion but just about anyone can recognize love when they see it.) At one point in our conversation—when Mark was describing what he called one of the "dramatic moments" (actually, a difficult point) during Tammi's treatment for breast cancer—he summed up their relationship by saying, "We do these things together."

It had been 18 months, rather than the usual 12 months, when Tammi went in for her "annual" mammogram at age 49. "I was having a little bit of discomfort in my breast, but I have the Ashkenazi gene—the fibrocystic breast thing—and they're always hurting. I could never do a good self-exam because I always would say, 'I think … hmm. I think … hmm. I *think* it's lumpy in the same place where it was the last month.' That was the best that I could tell. I went for my mammogram and told them that it hurt a little. I had just come back from New Jersey from a niece's bat mitzvah. I called up Friday morning, and they were able to get me in on Friday afternoon.

"The technician took about 30 seconds to do the films. She said, 'You can get dressed and go home. We'll call you.' Before I left, something made me ask, 'Does everything look okay?' She looked at me like I was nuts and said, 'Everything looks fine, but if you want to wait in the waiting room, the radiologist is still here and I'll have him take a quick look.'"

Tammi chuckled and rolled her eyes. "I'm sitting in the waiting room and feeling like a total hypochondriac. About 10 minutes later, I hear the radiologist say, 'Do you want to bring Ms. Bornstein back here?' So I go back to his office and he's looking at my prior films with a magnifying glass. He says, 'I want to get another film of your left breast.' It shocked me. For years, they had always done an extra film on that side. In fact, that's probably what surprised me—that the technician didn't automatically take another film.

"I said, 'Oh, that doesn't surprise me.' I was not really concerned. The radiologist said, 'Let me show you what I'm looking at. It could be that we're doing digital films now. In retrospect, we don't know if we're looking at something new. That's why I'm looking at your old films with a magnifying glass to try and see if what I'm seeing now is what I saw before. This is the area that concerns me.'"

Tammi wrinkled her brow and frowned. "At this point I start getting a little nervous. He tells the tech that he wants a magnified view, and he asks if the ultrasound machine is still on. So she does the film and says, 'Don't get dressed again, just in case he needs something else.' Sure enough he wants an ultrasound. He does the ultrasound and shows me what he's looking at.

"He takes my hand and he says, 'I'm sorry to tell you this at 5 o'clock on a Friday afternoon, but this needs to come out somehow. If this were my daughter, or if you were my wife, I would be telling you the same thing. There's a 75% chance that this is nothing. We're seeing a cluster of microcalcifications. From 25% to 30% of the time, it's something, but the rest of the time it turns out to be absolutely nothing. If it is something, what we're dealing with is ductal carcinoma *in situ,* which is very easily treated with 100% cure rate with a lumpectomy and a course of tamoxifen.'

"I asked the radiologist if he would call Mark to explain to him what he had told me. I knew that I would get home and wouldn't be able to explain it to Mark and he would have all these questions for me and I'd get confused, especially with the weekend and all."

The radiologist also contacted Tammi's gynecologist the following Monday at about noon, who, in turn, called Tammi and recommended a surgeon. "The gynecologist told me that he was going to call the surgeon and to wait about 10 minutes and then call the surgeon's office … When I called, they knew who I was and scheduled an appointment for the following day."

When I heard how rapidly she had gotten an appointment with a surgeon, I blurted out, "Wow!" and joked that only attorneys are treated that deferentially by physicians.

Tammi used to practice law but, after being diagnosed with breast cancer, she decided to change direction with her career. "Most recently I was doing transaction, corporate, and estate planning. One of the things I decided—one of the *first* decisions I made when I was diagnosed—was that the *last* thing I want to do is estate planning. I don't want to talk to people about their deaths—planning for their deaths.

"My passion has always been dogs. My animals put a smile on my face more than anything else, so I'd like to see what I could do to take that passion and use it for the common good … I could do volunteer work. I'd like to do pet therapy but you can't get insurance. It is prohibitive. All of the organizations that I could do it through and have insurance, you have to be a volunteer. I go to the Cancer Wellness Center. One of the things they don't have is dogs or animals to help people feel better.

"Also, I was reading the *Parade* section in the Sunday [*Chicago*] *Tribune* and there was a feature article on health insurance and how cancer patients cannot get insurance. One woman—who had for years been working and paying the cancer premiums to her employer—got down-sized and then diligently paid COBRA for 18 months. She had not been able to find a job in this economy. She had a recurrence of breast cancer and she doesn't have insurance. She clearly needs treatment, but she can't afford it.

"The article was replete with stories about individuals who either didn't have insurance, were underinsured, or who were denied insurance. After reading this article, I was thinking of forming a foundation or becoming an employee of an existing foundation so that I could do something to help people with health insurance problems. It just struck such a chord.

"In Illinois, Governor Ryan is staying executions because of flaws in the system." Tammi shook her head. "There have been so many medical advances, but they're denying people treatment because they don't have insurance. If they can't afford it, they're being denied access to a medical treatment. Basically, you're handing down *death* sentences. Governor Ryan and the medical insurance system are *handing down death sentences to these people*." Tammi's voice reflected her righteous indignation. She paused to calm herself, before adding, "I'm wondering if there's an opportunity for me to do something along those lines.

"I'm looking to make a positive impact for a common good. I want to change my whole focus. It's my way of dealing with my diagnosis. A psychologist I talked to told me that I have to find the reason for this, to come to terms with why this happened to me, and to find meaning in it. Maybe the way I can find meaning in it is to create some common good, something positive. Of course, Mark played an important role and helped me in this journey."

Mark nodded and continued their story: "I knew she was going in for a test. She kept me abreast—let me think of another word—she kept me *apprised* of what was going on. In my profession, I have to be a hopeful person. I am a psychologist and half my practice is with hospital patients and 10% of them die [while in the hospital]. I work at a hospital for catastrophically ill people, so I often try to find something to be hopeful about. The way that it was presented to me, I thought, it's probably okay. A 75% chance that it's okay, a 25% chance that it isn't okay, but if it isn't okay, there's a 100% chance that it's going to be fine. I can handle that, because I see a lot worse than that every day. I don't fight the numbers. Based on what they thought it was, it was 100% curable and you go with it. But then we had to deal with the tough stuff. One of the toughest things was telling the kids."

Tammi and Mark decided to postpone telling their children until more precise information was available, which meant waiting for the biopsy results. Tammi continued their story: "Mark came with me to see the surgeon, who checked out everything. He looked at the films and confirmed the radiologist's impression and suggested a stereotactic core biopsy. He said, 'I could do surgery, but if it's something suspicious, we're going to go in and operate again. Stereotactic biopsies are very, very accurate.'"

For a stereotactic breast biopsy, the patient lies on her abdomen with her breast hanging through a hole in the table. Using either three-dimensional computerized or digital imaging techniques, the radiologist pinpoints the worrisome area and then obtains cylindrical tissue samples with a vacuum-assisted needle biopsy device. This approach for obtaining a breast biopsy is particularly helpful when there is a nonpalpable mass that is visible by routine mammography or when there is a cluster of suspicious calcifications.

I was scheduled to have a stereotactic biopsy because of a small, but *palpable*, mass that developed microcalcifications; however, the radiologist to whom I was referred for the stereotactic biopsy—a man who was considered *"the very best"* at reading mammograms—assured me that I didn't need a biopsy. I left his office feeling embarrassed and ashamed of myself for wasting his time. It turned out that his disregard of a palpable mass with new microcalcifications was to delay my diagnosis of breast cancer by eight months.

It was only because I made an appointment with a new gynecologist for an unrelated symptom—irregular and heavy periods that had, in fact, been trivialized by my previous gynecologist—that I had a biopsy eight months later. (I am trying not to be shrill, but forgive me if I am.) My new gynecologist was Dr. Beth Engelsgjerd, a friend from medical school, to whom I invariably referred patients when they asked for a woman gynecologist. Just as invariably, the women thanked me for the referral and raved about how much they *adored* Dr. Engelsgjerd.

During her thorough breast exam, she palpated my breast mass and blurted out, "What's this?"

I answered, "Oh, it's just a little thing that we've been following for a while. Dr. Dismissive [not his real name] reviewed the films last October and said it's nothing."

Beth said, "Hmmm. Well, okay."

She called me about two weeks later and said, "Deb, I've been worrying about that little breast mass ever since I saw you. I really think you need to have it biopsied. Will you do that for me?"

I said, "Sure, if you think it needs it."

"Actually, I want you to have it biopsied right away."

"Well, okay."

"Do you promise?" Beth said.

"I promise."

Had I not promised Beth that I would have a biopsy done, I am fairly certain that I would have further postponed the procedure. The surgeon whom I consulted is a very, very good friend and one of the best surgeons I have ever worked with; however, he said, after doing an exam and reviewing the x-ray studies, "Debbey, I really don't think this is anything. Why don't we give it six months."

Apologetically I said, "I know I'm probably wasting everybody's time, but I promised Beth that I would have it biopsied."

It turned out that I wasn't wasting anyone's time. I had intermediate grade ductal carcinoma *in situ,* which extended to the margins, requiring a second surgical procedure to achieve negative margins. A quarter of my right breast was eventually removed.

Two and a half years later, I called Dr. Dismissive to tell him what had happened. I was not angry or accusatory. He said that he was sorry, and I chose (and still choose) to believe that he meant it. I said, "No apology is necessary. I just thought you might want to review the films for educational purposes."

Tammi had a stereotactic biopsy three days later (on Friday) and received the pathology results by telephone the following Monday. "I asked if it was ductal carcinoma *in situ* and he said, 'No, it's a little bit more than that, but it's low grade. A portion of it is infiltrating.' So we went to schedule surgery, but his first date available for surgery conflicted with our 12-year-old son Adam's school musical. I said, 'Omigod, I want to get this thing out,' but he said, 'It's low grade. It can wait.'

"So we waited. My brother, who's a pediatrician in Boston, said, 'Don't rush into surgery. Get your team together first.' The surgeon said, 'No one is going to talk to you until you have all of the information from the pathology report.' My brother still said, 'Get your team together. I don't want you to have surgery.'

"At first, we were running around trying to find an oncologist and a radiologist, but the surgeon was right. We could barely find an oncologist who would talk to us without having all the information. We eventually found an oncologist who reminded us of Marcus Welby and who talked to us without even having the full pathology report and gave us his recommendations based on what he saw. We even went to see him in his office where he examined me and talked about options. May 14 [2004] was the surgery. The pathology results came in within a week of the surgery. Ductal carcinoma, 1.1 cm, grade 2. Margins clear. Sentinel nodes—four nodes negative. Stage I. Originally, they weren't thinking of chemo, but …" Tammi shrugged and looked at Mark.

Mark continued their story. "They said that chemotherapy would increase the survival rate by 10%. A computer program we used increased the survival from 85% to 95%. You wanted an 'A,' right, Tammi?" Mark slid his arm around Tammi's shoulder and they both laughed.

Tammi had four cycles of Adriamycin® and Cytoxan® followed by external beam radiation therapy. At the time that she and Mark walked in the Chicago 3-Day, Tammi had received her last chemotherapy treatment on August 4, 2004, which was just three weeks before the walk. She was still quite bald. The prospect that she would go bald had *initially* seemed to be the major concern for their children.

Mark continued. "The only other experience they had with breast cancer was with their playmates. There's a family, the Fiorentinis, with two boys. The older boy is Adam's age; the younger boy is our 10-year-old daughter Abby's age. They were friends, and we were friends with their parents. The mother died of breast cancer pretty quickly—a snow-balling, bad course. So their experience with breast cancer was that it kills you. We were basically trying to wait to tell them, until we had to tell them … I believe Mother's Day was coming up and we talked to the rabbi, who said, 'Tell them. Don't worry. You don't want to keep that a secret on Mother's Day.'

"We practiced and practiced. I think we handled it pretty well." Mark looked at Tammi to see if she agreed, and she nodded. Mark continued. "The kids handled that part of it well. We told them that there are two types of breast cancer. One type is the kind that Mrs. Fiorentini had, and that kind can kill you. There's another type where you get some surgery and cut it out, and afterwards you're fine.

"So Adam said, 'Who's got that type? Abby?'" Tammi and Mark looked at each other and laughed. "I said, 'No, your mother has that type.' We explained to them that she may have to have some treatment and may lose her hair. 'Omigod,' they said, 'Don't let our friends see that!'

"We thought they were dealing with it well, but Adam's having some sort of night terrors. He's having a lot of fear so we're trying to help him out. He's a boy and not as open with his emotions. He's getting counseling and he's doing better."

Tammi continued their story: "Adam had heard that men can get breast cancer. He thought that if one person in the family got cancer, it meant that other people in the family would get cancer, like an infectious process. He had pointed this out to a very good friend of ours. She's the mother of a friend of his and she is like a second mother to him. She calls Adam her third son and we call Ben our second son. She jokes that she has custody of him every other weekend when he sleeps at her house. I took Adam to the pediatrician and he told the pediatrician that he was worried about what I was going to look like without hair. The pediatrician told him, 'I'll bet your mother is wondering, too.' I was getting my head shaved that day—my hair was falling out in clumps—and I said, 'You're not going to have to wait long to find out.' After Adam talked to the pediatrician, he slept better that night.

"They told us it would start coming out beginning day 14, and then it would come out with increasing acceleration. I tell people that NASA couldn't have timed a fuel burn with more accuracy." Mark and Tammi looked at each other, nodded, and laughed again. Together they described a "shower scene that would rival the scene in *Psycho*" when Tammi's hair started coming out in clumps. Unbeknownst to Tammi, when she stepped out of the shower wet globs of hair were sticking to her body. Mark attempted to dry her off with a towel before she had a chance to realize the dramatic hair loss but the terry cloth towel only served to smear the wisps of hair; however, just as he got her dried off, she remembered that she hadn't rinsed the conditioner out of her hair and told Mark that she needed to return to the shower. Mark asked, "Why did you put on conditioner?" and Tammi answered, "I don't know."

Tammi said, "I'm losing my hair but, in my own mind, I still had to put conditioner on my hair. I got back in the shower and more hair is coming out as I was rinsing out the conditioner. We had to go through the whole thing all over again. It had been coming out in increasing amounts, but that day it was coming out so much. The toupee in the bottom of my shower was getting bigger and bigger. When it had first started coming out, I called Mark over to show him all the hair that was in the bottom of the shower. His first reaction was, 'Well, we knew this was going to happen.'"

Tammi smiled at Mark, who smiled sheepishly and nodded. He said, "That was a bad response."

Tammi said, still smiling, "That was a real bad response, but he regrouped and said, 'That was a bad response.'"

Mark shrugged and said, "That was when I knew I wasn't perfect."

He may not have been perfect, but it wasn't for lack of trying. During her chemotherapy Mark pitched in to help Tammi with the household duties. Mark said, "It reminded me how time-consuming and tiring it is to take care of household duties. I have these husbands [his patients] complaining that their wives don't do anything. I can tell them now ..."

Tammi also got help from an unexpected source. "People whom I didn't know very well have stepped up to the plate. One woman in Lincolnshire, who was a neighbor—actually the mother of one of Abby's very good friends; I can't say we ever went out together—took it upon herself to call and ask me for a list of our friends. She coordinated a meal schedule. When she called me, I couldn't even return her phone call for two or three days, because I was so choked up. I asked her, 'Why are you doing this?' and she said, 'That's what people do. When someone needs help, you help. That's why we were put on this earth, to help other people.'" Tammi's voice cracked, and she paused to compose herself before continuing.

"I'd like to think that I would have done the same but, before this happened to me, I honestly don't know if I would have. This whole process has made me a better person. Life gets in the way. I don't know if I was really the best friend I could have been to people. Like Mark's friends. Not one of Mark's friends has called."

Mark nodded and said, "My best friend called once after about three months. I believe that people think they should be saying something wonderful—just the right thing—and when they can't, they don't know what to do and they get embarrassed. They don't call, and then it's a long time and they get more embarrassed, and they don't call. I've been let down. In the emotional area, I may be considered the senior man among the group because I'm older and because of what I do. That doesn't excuse it, but I'm trying to rationalize their behavior ... I went to a support group meeting, but I spent the whole time trying to figure out how to say something supportive of the other people ... I think I'm doing okay. Exercise has been my antidepressant."

Mark turned to Tammi and asked her how she was feeling. She answered that she was doing fine. Mark said, "I was concerned that she might do some damage."

Tammi repeated, "I'm fine, but tomorrow may be different."

Mark added, "Tammi takes it one rest stop at a time."

I reassured her that being swept to camp was not a sign of failure and urged her to take it easy. Sliding into my familiar (but, no doubt, annoying) role as older sister, I reminded her that chemotherapy stresses all systems and that it was wise not to demand too much of her body.

"I'll sweep in if necessary. My reason for being here is that I need to stare down this disease. I just need to say, 'It's not going to win.'"

Mark and Tammi finished Day 1 without being swept to camp. Beginning in Kenosha, Wisconsin, they walked the full 19.1 miles through Pleasant Prairie, Winthrop Harbor, Zion, Beach Park, and Waukegan, ending the day at Camp One in North Chicago.

For me, that Friday night was one of the most memorable of all the camps. In addition to the usual dinnertime and evening activities, we were treated to a surprise performance by the North Chicago Hi-Stepper Drill Team and Drum Corps. (I say "surprised" because it wasn't on the Chicago Camp One schedule card that we were given as we finished the day's route.) About 20 young people performed, including three young men who played drums and a fourth who blew a whistle to signal the beginning of precision marching and dance routines. The remainder were young women, most of whom appeared to be in high school. A girl about 11 or 12 years old was in the center of the first row. Despite being the youngest, she was just as snappy and talented as the others. It was hard to keep from paying her the most attention because of her enthusiasm and smile. (Inexplicably, when a well-disciplined marching band takes the field at half-time at a football game, I always get tight-throated. Watching the North Chicago Hi-Stepper Drill Team and Drum Corps affected me the same way.)

Tammi was also able to finish the 23.4-mile route on Day 2 through Lake Bluff, Lake Forest Highwood, Highland Park, Genco, Hubbardwood, Winnetka, Kenilworth, Evanston, Wilmette, and Skokie. The temperature stayed in the 60s all day, but the weather was gray and uninspiring, misting just enough to dampen enthusiasm. Still, Tammi finished.

Unfortunately, soon after arriving in camp on Day 2, she became ill and had to be transported to the hospital for hydration. We three had planned to meet again but, when I reached Mark by cell phone, they were at home. Tammi was doing much better but, clearly, they wouldn't be walking Day 3. I promised Mark that I would call them the next day when I learned the details of Closing Ceremonies.

On Day 3, Tammi was feeling much better and was able to take her place in the Survivors' Circle for Closing Ceremonies. Among the group of women holding hands in the Survivors' Circle was Robin Goldfarb, who was not a breast cancer survivor; however, Robin's friend, Joshua Markus, was carrying the 3-Day flag for Closing Ceremonies and Robin had been asked to fill in, probably for Tammi, before they knew she would, indeed, be able to participate. Robin and I had walked together for a few miles on Day 2.

Robin was walking with Joshua Markus, whose wife, Liza Markus, had died on May 6, 2004, following a two-and-a-half-year battle with breast cancer. Liza was a few weeks shy of her 34th birthday when she died. Robin and Liza grew up together in New York, and Robin had known Joshua since he and Liza started dating. In 1998, when Joshua and Liza got married, Robin was in their wedding party.

Robin said that she and Liza had been friends since they were 11 years old. "We were practically the same age. My birthday was a week and a half after hers. We were very close. Liza was all about helping other people. She worked in Chicago at a place where they help under-privileged people turn their lives around: get jobs, get back on their feet, find housing, that sort of thing. I gave the eulogy at her funeral. I had to do it. My dad is one of the people who always gives eulogies at funerals. He's just known for doing that, and I had to carry on the tradition. We knew each other for so long that I felt like I had to offer the eulogy—for me, for Josh, for Liza.

"One of the things I said in the eulogy is that she helped so many people and that I felt like I had to keep her life meaningful by doing something that made a difference—whatever I could do to keep her spirit alive.

It would make me feel better. Maybe it was selfish, but every time I would do something like that I would be thinking about her and that would keep her spirit alive." Tears filled Robin's eyes and we walked in silence for a while.

"On the way home from the funeral, Josh saw a poster for the 3-Day event and told me about it at the shiva. In Jewish tradition, right after the funeral, you sit shiva for seven days. Families come to offer their condolences and you say a prayer. I didn't really decide right away because, obviously, the next few weeks were very difficult. The funeral was in New York, where we grew up, and I went to Chicago the next week for the memorial service. Joshua and Liza lived in Chicago and I was living in New York. I decided that I also needed to do the memorial service in Chicago and give my eulogy again for those friends and family members. No one was going to be there from her younger life, from her childhood.

"I had pretty much decided by the time I got to Chicago that I would do the walk with Josh. I wasn't sure if it was something that he wanted to do by himself. So I said, 'I would really like to do the walk with you,' and he said, 'That would be great,' and here we are. "It's been great, but it's been tough, too—especially the Opening Ceremonies. We stayed in Kenosha on Thursday night and that was one of the more emotional times of this whole weekend because we just talked about Liza a lot and remembered and reminisced. We were both getting upset, but I think it's also been very cathartic. Between the two of us, we raised, including corporate matches, over $20,000, so we feel like we've really made a difference, and maybe we can prevent some other families and friends from going through the same thing that we've just been through."

Robin described how walking a few miles in the morning before work helped her deal with the almost-paralyzing grief. "One of my best friends lives in my building, and she would come with me in the mornings before work for a couple of miles. It was really helpful to get out of bed, go to work, and talk to people about it. Even though my mind wasn't necessarily focused on work or the relevance of why I needed to be at work, I was still getting there and doing my job—just showing people that I felt like I needed to do something to make a difference. It really helped me to get past that difficult part.

"My two grandmothers passed away a few years ago. I was pretty upset, but I don't remember it hitting me like Liza's death did. I think, in part, it was because of her age … I was in her wedding party; she was supposed to be in mine. There were so many things that we had talked about doing. When we were little girls, we talked about the future and what we were going to do together when we got older. Liza is just such an amazing person."

When I pointed out to Robin that she had used the present tense, she looked pained, and I immediately wished I hadn't mentioned her mistake. I tried to apologize for my insensitivity by describing how I had used the present tense for months after my husband died. In fact, I still have what I call "pronoun slippage," especially when talking about my children. (I frequently say "our children.")

Robin finished her thought, despite my interruption. "Liza was one of those people that you aspire to be like. Everyone she touched was so moved by her."

Robin is a computer technical consultant with Sun Microsystems. Liza's death has affected the way that Robin views her career. "I used to be very into work. I wanted to meet someone, get married, and have kids, but work was always a priority. For better or worse, now I go to work and say, 'It's just a job.' Josh and I have been talking along the way. We've had the rain, and we've had all these obstacles along the way, but we keep telling ourselves that it's not about the destination, it's about the journey. In the last couple of months, I've gotten that it's about really living your life. Spending time with your friends. Spending time with your family. Your job is there to give you the means to do that.

"That's a completely different attitude than I've had in the past. Liza's given me all these things, and she's still giving me all these things ..." Robin's voice trailed off, and tears came to her eyes again. She said quietly, "Even though she's not physically here, she's still here. That's probably why I used the present tense earlier."

———

For Closing Ceremonies, Joshua Markus was asked to carry the 3-Day flag in the Survivors' Circle. He was wearing dark sunglasses and appeared calm and composed as he moved toward the stationary flagpole, encircled by six women holding hands, including his friend, Robin Goldfarb, and Tammi Bornstein. On cue, Joshua left the circle, and he and one of the 3-Day staff detached the banner from the flagstaff and fastened it to the flagpole halyard. Joshua raised the flag and stepped back. As he gazed up at the flag, a tear slid down his cheek from behind the dark glasses. I felt like I had been hit in the chest.

I knew that this man would never get over the death of his young wife. Not ever. I knew that any person who quips that time heals everything has not watched a loved one die from cancer. (Case in point: While writing the opening paragraphs of this chapter, I cried as hard as I've ever cried about my husband's death.) When I saw Joshua's sadness, I hoped with all my heart that his 3-Day experience had brought him a measure of comfort.

———

I was reminded of a conversation I had with the woman beside me on the bus ride to the Chicago Opening Ceremonies. The woman's name was Ilana Balaban and she spoke with an accent. She was 64 years old and was walking in her fifth 3-Day event. A friend of hers who was a breast cancer survivor was visiting from Israel, so Ilana was torn between walking in the 3-Day again this year or spending time with her friend. Ilana said, "My friend insisted that I walk because it is a mitzvah. Do you know the word?"

"Like in bar mitzvah?"

"Yes, it is the same word, but mitzvah is also the Hebrew word for a good deed, a worthy deed. My friend says that walking in the 3-Day is a mitzvah."

"Your friend is right," I said. "It is a very worthy deed."

Participating in a 3-Day event by raising money and walking is a worthy deed, but so is volunteering for one of the 3-Day crew teams. There are three main divisions: Camp Teams, Road Teams, and Health Services Teams. There are nine labor divisions of Camp Teams with duties like loading gear, serving meals, managing the information tent, setting up the campsite, checking in walkers at the end of the route, and directing vehicles to designated parking areas. The Road Teams deliver ice and water to the Pit Stops, patrol the route by bicycle or motorcycle (sometimes being stationed at heavy-traffic intersections), set up and run the Pit Stops and lunch stops, mark the route with directional signs, and drive vans that sweep walkers with fatigue or medical problems.

To be on the Health Services Team, volunteers must have insurance, licensure, and certification in the event state. In other words, this team is comprised of doctors, physician assistants, nurses, and emergency medical technicians. The other Health Services Teams are Medical Transport and Sports Medicine (athletic trainers, physical therapists, and chiropractors).

Other year-round volunteer opportunities include answering questions about the 3-Day by telephone, leading training walks, mentoring other walkers, helping at expos, assisting at orientation sessions, and helping at Opening and Closing Ceremonies.

Cathy Petry, 56, was a four-year survivor of breast cancer in 1999 when she participated in her first 3-Day event as a walker. She has participated on volunteer crews every year since then. "In 2000 and 2001, I crewed one event; in 2002, I expanded and did two walks; last year [2003], I did seven events; this year, I'm doing eight. I get six weeks of vacation, so that's how I use my vacation.

"I know people who have walked and then crewed. After they crew, they say, 'I'm going back to walking. This is hard work.' It can be hard work, but it's so much fun. It's what you make of it. You get with a group of people and start to have fun with them. What *I* like is that I get to meet the same people year after year. I wish I had the stamina to do the Gear and Tent Crew because everyone has a blast with that one. They have *such* a good time. Last year in San Francisco, as crew, our tent was right on the end near the Gear and Tent trucks. They have to stay up until the last piece of gear is claimed and they're back at 4:30 in the morning to start loading up again. It's hard work, yeah, but it's worth it. Besides, even the worst day in crew is better than the best day at chemotherapy."

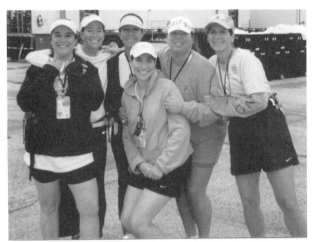

Debby Padzensky, far right, with Ron's Ribbons

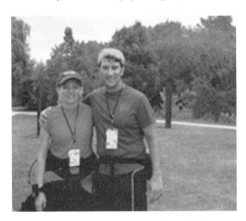

Robin Goldfarb and Joshua Markus

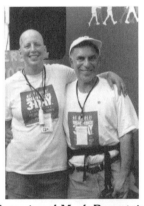

Tammi and Mark Bornstein

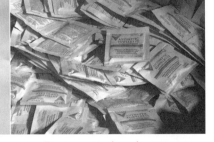

If your URINE
is darker than this
paper, YOU
NEED TO DRINK
MORE FLUIDS!!!

Sign on porta-potty in Chicago   *Porta-potty hand wipes*

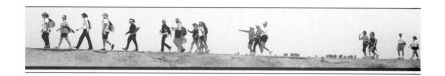

Chapter 6

Twin Cities

September 10, September 11, and September 12, 2004

Bunion surgery vies with hemorrhoid surgery for being the least glamorous of surgical procedures. This may be part of the reason why those afflicted often postpone treatment until they begin to walk funny. Bunions (on the big toe bone) and hemorrhoids (on the tail end) differ in how they cause people to walk funny.

Inflamed bunions cause people to limp, sometimes leaning backwards with their weight on their heels. On the other end, painful hemorrhoids cause people to walk deliberately, sometimes with their backs slightly arched. After their operations, both sets of patients continue to walk funny, at least for a while; however, the telltale signs of a recent hemorrhoidectomy (hemorrhoid removal) are under wraps, while those of a bunionectomy (bunion removal) are in plain sight. Furthermore, depending on the extent of surgery, bunionectomy patients sometimes wear a cast-like boot for weeks, maybe even for a few months. (If you're squeamish, skip the next two paragraphs.)

My bunion surgery involved not only shaving off the knob-like overgrowth of bone on the side of the big toe (the bunion itself), but also removing wafers of bone from the first and second metatarsals with insertion of two wires to hold everything in place during healing. After accomplishing their job, the wires had to be yanked out. This last step took place in the doctor's office, while I was fully awake. Allow me to elaborate. (This is the *final warning* for squeamish readers!)

The surgeon first anesthetized the skin overlying the wires by injecting Xylocaine® with a needle. Next, he made a little cut in the skin and, using what looked like a pair of needle-nosed pliers, fished around until he found the tips of the wires. Once seized upon, the wires evidently wanted to stay put in their dark, cozy tunnels among the bones and, like recalcitrant earthworms, only burrowed deeper when the doctor tried to extract them. The wire-yanking had been described to me as being "a piece of cake"; however, by the time it was done, both the orthopedic surgeon and I were drenched with sweat, glaring at each other. (I declined his offer to take the wires home as souvenirs.)

If the surgery had been done in summer 1997, when it was originally planned, bone removal and the business with the wires would not have been necessary; however, that was the summer that my father was diagnosed with a malignant brain tumor, and getting my foot fixed was postponed. Still, a few years later, when my foot started intermittently going to sleep, I became concerned that the drifting bones might be compressing a blood vessel or a nerve, or both, and that irreversible damage might be afoot. I finally had the surgery in early 2001, nearly four years after the original scheduling.

The procedure did resolve the problem with my foot going to sleep but, for a long time after the surgery (and the wire-ferreting episode), my foot continued to hurt, although, admittedly, in a different way than it had before, causing me to shift my weight to my heels to avoided pushing off the balls of my feet. I plodded, which is not to be confused with walking deliberately, although the two might be impossible to distinguish.

By the time my foot mended, my compensatory, backward-leaning gait had become habit. This caused balance problems, of course, particularly when walking on uneven surfaces or hiking in the mountains. I developed a fear of falling and began to walk more slowly. In retrospect, this uneasiness with going forward was a metaphor for something deeper. The doctor may have fixed my foot, but he couldn't fix my shuffling approach to life.

Two and a half years after the bunion surgery, an incident exposed how timid I had become. August 7, 2003, was the four-year anniversary of my husband's death. My best friend anticipated that I might need a boost, so she invited me to go to a women's professional basketball game. When my son, 18 years old at the time, learned that I had accepted the invitation, he was astonished. He said, "Mom, I didn't think you'd ever do anything like that again. It makes me glad to see you getting back to your old self."

Until then, it hadn't occurred to me that my children had noticed my hesitancy. This troubled me since, as their mother, it was my job to *clear* a path, not just creep along, flinching at shadows. Something had to be done.

On a whim—but not seriously thinking that I would actually do it— I had previously registered for the 2004 Arizona 3-Day; however, within two days of the basketball game, I registered for the nine other 2004 Breast Cancer 3-Day events. My goal was to prove to my kids that I hadn't turned into a weenie.

Later came the idea of interviewing other walkers for a book. This meant that I would be walking 600 miles in 10 cities over a three-month period. It sounded kind of nutty and, from the looks people gave me, I'm reasonably certain that many of them thought I had slipped a cog or two.

There were times—many times, in fact—that I wondered if my plans were grandiose and if I had, indeed, developed a lithium deficiency. (Lithium carbonate is the drug that is used to treat symptoms of manic-depressive disorder, with signs like grandiosity and poor judgment.)

Besides the odd looks and self-doubt, there were other stumbling blocks, not the least of which was, literally, the physical part of moving forward. My 52-year-old feet—after running 11 full marathons in their 20s and early 30s—didn't appreciate the return to asphalt streets. The previous bunion surgery didn't help matters. I tried coaxing them along with all sorts of things: taking analgesics and anti-inflammatories, doing stretching exercises, changing the training surface, and switching shoes. I finally consulted a sports podiatrist for custom-fitted orthotics, which helped immeasurably.

Next, my college-aged children were undergoing some major (and positive) transitions in their lives, which required my attention, expertise, and presence with a checkbook. Lastly, and most difficult to resolve, I began to question the validity of the project itself (do we really need another book about breast cancer survivorship?) and my abilities to do justice to the task (will I be able to effectively order the narratives of the people who share their stories?). Still, using what my fiancé called the "bludgeon method," I trudged on.

Fast-forward to the afternoon of September 10, 2004, Day 1 of the Twin Cities event. This was a little past the halfway mark of the goal to walk all 600 miles of the 2004 3-Day events. Boston, New York City, Washington, D.C., Michigan, and Chicago were behind me; San Diego, Los Angeles, San Francisco, and Arizona were ahead of me. I had gotten tight-throated and sometimes cried in six Opening Ceremonies and five Closing Ceremonies, camped in schoolyards and on playgrounds, ate meals while sitting on folding chairs under tents and on pieces of pasteboard in parking lots, showered in semi-trucks, and napped on the bare ground and in airport chairs. I had become friends with two people who treated me like family. I had heard stories that fed my soul. Since beginning the project, I had also spent many hours "alone" while on airplanes, in cabs, on airport shuttles, in restaurants, on buses, in hotel rooms, and on the pavement walking. Yet, it was on this particular day, in Richfield, Minnesota, that something remarkable happened.

Opening Ceremonies that morning had been at Canterbury Park in Shakopee, southwest of Minneapolis. From Shakopee, we had headed northeast, crossed the Minnesota River, and walked along trails overlooking the Minnesota River Valley. Day 1's route was 22.5 miles and went through Eden Prairie, Richfield, and Hopkins, and ended in St. Louis Park. It was a partly cloudy day, in the 70s, and many of the miles were on some of the interlinking park system trails. At lunch, I had met two interesting women from Iowa, and we had walked together for the early part of the afternoon.

But the breakthrough occurred later that afternoon, while I was walking "alone" beside a park where cheering friends and family members of the walkers had gathered. As I waved and shouted thank you, it suddenly occurred to me that my old gait was back. I was taking big steps. I was pushing off with the balls of my feet. I was no longer afraid of falling. For the first time in *years*, the road ahead brimmed with opportunity. I laughed out loud, tears running down my cheeks, profoundly grateful. It felt good to be back on my feet.

The original intent of this book was to explore cancer's convolutions through the stories of those affected. Sharing the voluntary journey of a 3-Day event turned out to be a compelling context to explore the involuntary journey of breast cancer. What I didn't anticipate was how life-changing the event would be for so many of the participants, me included. At roughly the half-way point of the project, in Richfield, Minnesota, it sank in.

———————

The women from Iowa whom I had met earlier that day—before the Richfield realization—were sisters-in-law Jo Ann Merfeld and Pat Weiss. Jo Ann was married to Pat's younger brother, Pete, but the women interacted more like sisters (or good friends) than in-laws. This was particularly apparent when Pat bragged about her younger sister-in-law. "Jo Ann was raised on a dairy farm in Kentucky, only to decide that she was going to get off that dairy farm some day. And she did and went to Purdue. Now, she's senior vice president of a bank. She's very meticulous and researches everything. It was the same with her cancer."

Jo Ann Merfeld was 44 years old when her annual mammogram revealed an abnormality, which proved, by ultrasound, to be a fluid-filled cyst. "My PA [physician's assistant] called to tell me that the radiologist's report said that there was no evidence of cancer and that there was nothing to worry about. As I talked further to the PA, she said, 'There's no way to be 100% sure unless they do a biopsy. In order to have a definite diagnosis, we would need to send you to a surgeon.' She said there was no *medical* reason for me to worry, but I asked her what she would do, and she said, 'I'd do a biopsy. That would be the ultra-, ultra-cautious thing to do.'

"So she made an appointment for me with a surgeon in Mason City, Iowa, and I went in within a couple of days. Of course, my husband said, 'Would you like me to go with you?' and I said, 'There's no point in you going. They're just going to look at me, examine me, and then they'll probably schedule it,' but when I get there, of course, he [the surgeon] does the biopsy that day. For the cyst, he used a needle to pull out tons of greenish-looking fluid. He did a full exam and said that I had a lot of very fibrous tissue. He said, 'You know, I think there's a couple of other spots here that I'd like to also do needle biopsies on.' One was on the same side [as the fluid-filled cyst] and one was on the other side."

I asked Jo Ann if she was concerned that the "spots" might be cancer. She said, "I remember that it gave me pause, but I wasn't too worried ... I believe in finding out the facts and not jumping to conclusions or getting overly excited about something until I know what's going on. That's really how I approach problems ... At this point, we were just being overly careful, pretty much ... A week later, Pete and I go back [for an appointment with the surgeon] and he says that the results of the biopsies were inconclusive. 'What I would like to do is to go in and do a surgical biopsy and remove the lumps.'" Jo Ann and her sister-in-law, Pat, almost simultaneously looked at each other, raised their eyebrows, nodded their heads, and pressed their lips together.

"So then I had the surgical biopsies in two different places—one on one side; one on the other—both were in places that were not in the original process but were something that he had felt during the exam. Keep in mind, I had had a breast exam from the PA, as well, within the last month, so this surgeon was very thorough. He came out of surgery and told my husband that he was very sure that it was a [benign] cyst. I was supposed to go back the following Friday to have the stitches out and to get the formal [pathology] lab results, but they called me on Tuesday and said, 'You know, we're trying to rearrange the doctor's schedule. Would you mind coming in on Wednesday instead?' I said, 'Okay, that's fine.'

"So I'm going to see the surgeon, and my husband said, 'Do you want me to go with you?' and I said, 'Oh, no, they're just going to take out the stitches. There's no point in you taking off work. I'll be fine.'" Had she any idea that she was about to learn that she had breast cancer, she would have asked Pete to go along.

At diagnosis, in 2002, Jo Ann, her husband, Pete, and their sons Greg, 14, and Jason, 10, lived in Charles City, Iowa. Jo Ann's imaging studies, needle biopsies, and surgical biopsies were done in Mason City, 30 miles away from where she and her family lived. She had driven that particular stretch of highway scores of times during the years that she was pursuing her master's degree in business from Drake University through the Iowa Communications Network distance learning program at the community college.

In 1994, when she started the master's program, Jo Ann was working full-time in the Operations Department at a bank and her youngest son was only three years old. Still, she completed the master's program on schedule. Her upbringing, no doubt, had something to do with her perseverance.

Jo Ann was reared on a dairy farm in Kentucky and knew about hard physical labor. "We milked cows, and I did most of the milking. We raised corn for feed, and we raised tobacco for our cash crop. It was all family-worked. In high school, I had a job in town at a drug store. I went to work after school; then I came home and milked. On Saturdays, I milked; then I went to work; then I came home and milked again. I milked on Sunday morning before we went to church. It was a normal life, as far as I knew. Cows had to be milked ... We hoed tobacco. I drove a tractor while my father and two younger brothers loaded hay. There were only two things—because I was a girl—that I didn't have to do. One was pitch hay and the other was fork manure. I had to do everything else. I have no idea why my father picked those two things, because I did a lot of hard work.

"We didn't have a flush toilet until I was in seventh grade. An out-house. A slop jar. Do you know what those are?" Jo Ann looked at me and chuckled. "We had a wood-burning stove, and we got an indoor bathroom when the farm was paid for. When there was no mortgage, we started. My dad put in a bathroom and we put in a furnace. It was a pretty simple existence out of necessity.

"My dad's philosophy was that it was the parents' responsibility to teach their children to work and to take care of themselves, and he did that pretty well ... Dad was doing what he thought was the right thing, of course, but I had always known that it was not the kind of life that I wanted for myself. I didn't want to work that hard, and I wanted to be able to do some things that were enjoyable."

Jo Ann's first respite from her father's Kentucky farm came during the summer between her junior and senior years in high school when she was offered a slot at a national science training program at Purdue University based on her entrance and placement exam. "I studied at the vet school for two months, and I paid for it myself. I decided to go back there after I graduated ... I knew that I was going to college. My parents wanted me to go to college, but I was going to have to pay for it myself, so I worked the whole way through ...The first year I worked about 20 hours a week with a lady doing research on aging in rats ... Within two years of living on my own, I could qualify for student aid as an independent person, which allowed me to get more grants and loans and put myself through school."

Jo Ann graduated with a degree in agricultural economics. Her first job was in Iowa, working in sales for a farm supply company. Despite doing well, she didn't really enjoy sales. "During this period of time, I met my husband, and we got married. After two years, I changed jobs and started working at a local bank. I became an agricultural loan officer, which is more in line with what I wanted to do. So I was an ag loan officer during the 1980s, which was a terrible time for agriculture ... I handled the worst problem loans during that period of time—the litigation, the foreclosures."

I asked Jo Ann if, given her background, it was heartrending to deal with families who were struggling to keep their farms, and she said, "I had compassion for these people. I think the reason that I could stomach it was because my father always approached the farm as a business.

He loved it, but he knew it had to make money. I was the oldest and, even though I was a girl, he discussed the farm's finances with me. We would sit and talk and figure out the best business decision. When I was in high school, I studied the Internal Revenue Service code and did his income tax returns. I understood that you had to make money in order to support a family.

"I'd have to say that, during the 80s, a lot of farmers were coming to the realization that it was a business. It had to make money. If it didn't make money, you couldn't farm just for the sake of nostalgia. So I understood that part of it very well. I also knew what it was like to work very hard ... I still speak with almost all of my customers who went through really tough times. When I see them on the street, I talk to them; they ask me how my kids are. They're the people that I can still talk with." It was obvious that Jo Ann was proud of her ability to develop and maintain the respect of these farmers despite the situation's overwhelming potential for acrimony.

After completing her master's program in finance, the chairman of the bank asked her to apply for an administrative job in the Loan Department. When her bank merged with other banks, she took over loan administration work for all of the offices and was made senior vice president. For her entire career in banking, she has worked for the same chairman of the board. "He always supported me when I was young and green. He's always had a lot of confidence in me and has allowed me to make mistakes. I've worked for him almost 23 years. I worked more directly with him when the bank was much smaller. He's not retired, but he's not nearly as involved with the day-to-day activities as before, although I still have contact with him. If he wants to know something or wants something checked on, he calls me up."

Jo Ann's family's farm in Kentucky was sold shortly after her father died of a massive heart attack at age 49. "My mom was 47 when my dad died. I was out of college. Pete and I had been married a year and a half. My youngest brother was a senior in high school ... It was devastating for my mother, because my dad had always made all the decisions. She'd worked right beside him, but she had never decided anything. She just did whatever he said she should do. Taking care of the farm was way too much stress for her because she couldn't make the decisions. I was 700 miles away and I couldn't make them for her, and I wasn't going back there ... That farm was my dad's dream, not mine. It wasn't my mother's dream either."

Jo Ann was only 30 miles away from her husband and family when she learned the results of her biopsies, but she might as well have been 700 miles away. "So the surgeon comes in and says, 'We did find cancer in the right breast biopsy.'" Jo Ann laughed and added, "*That* was when I got worried ... The surgeon was talking to me about surgery and said,

'Do you want to call your husband?' I said, 'He's half an hour away, and by the time he gets here, it wouldn't be practical.'

"The surgeon walked out of the room, and I called my husband on the cell phone—he was expecting to take me out to lunch—and said, 'I have cancer.' He said, 'Do you want me to drive right over?' I'm thinking, No, then we'll have two cars in Mason City, and then we'll have to get them back, so I said, 'No, I'll just meet you at home. I have to have a lung x-ray and have some things done to prepare for this surgery. They want me to get the blood tests done right now. I'll let you know when I'm leaving.' He felt terrible that he had not been there with me, but it had been foolish of me, because I had said, 'Oh, no, you don't need to go.' I didn't cry that much until I got home. He felt awful. I think he still feels awful about that."

That night after dinner, Jo Ann and Pete sat down at the dining room table with their sons. "It was very hard to tell them, but we made the decision that we didn't want them hearing anything from anyone else that they didn't already know. We wanted them to know everything up front, and we didn't want them to feel like something was being kept from them. As a child, the worst thing is to hear adults talking and then thinking that something is worse than it really is because you're not being told. Sitting down and talking about something at the dining room table was not new. It's something that we'd always done, but this was a whole different matter.

"We told them that we found a lump in my breast, and we told them exactly where it was; told them that it was cancer; that we'd treat it; that it would be hard for everyone for a while, but that I'd be okay, because it was caught very early … They went off and had a talk with each other. After a few hours, they were back asking some questions. We answered every question completely, because they were old enough to comprehend the seriousness of it … I would do it again exactly the same way."

Jo Ann's cancer was an unexpected finding in the tissue adjacent to the wall of the benign cyst that was removed. The cancerous area was only 0.4 cm and had a single area of early invasion. This meant that Jo Ann was an excellent candidate for a wide local excision (lumpectomy or breast conservation treatment). She had a sentinel node biopsy, which was immediately followed by an axillary dissection, as a study participant.

The old wisdom held that all breast cancer patients benefited from an axillary node dissection. For locally advanced disease, this remains a defensible approach; however, for patients with early stage disease, scores of studies show that an axillary dissection offers no advantage over a sentinel lymph node biopsy for staging purposes.

To perform a sentinel node biopsy, the surgeon injects a tracer, such as isosulfan blue (a dye), at the tumor site (or in the tissue surrounding the previous biopsy site—the "tumor bed"). This tracer material enters the small lymphatic spaces and makes its way to the first lymph node(s) upstream from the breast—the sentinel nodes—which are the ones most likely to harbor metastatic cancer. These nodes are removed and examined microscopically. If the sentinel lymph nodes are negative for metastatic carcinoma, it's steady on; if not, it's back for more nodes.

Sentinel lymph node biopsies were first used in the mid-1990s but, like any new procedure, surgeons weren't allowed to simply read about it in a medical journal (or hear about it from an Internet-savvy patient) and then step up to the operating table and have at it. As with any new procedure, surgeons must first demonstrate proficiency. That's why Jo Ann's sentinel node biopsy was immediately followed by an axillary dissection. Her surgeon was in the proficiency demonstration period for doing sentinel lymph node biopsies and had enrolled Jo Ann in a study.

She continued. "So that was the Wednesday before Mother's Day, May 2002. A week later we went in for the results, and Pete went with me for that. When the doctor said, 'The lymph nodes are clear,' Pete broke down and cried. He said, 'I've never prayed for anything so hard in my life.' The breast cancer social worker was there also, and she said it must have been such a relief, because he just cried and cried. He was so relieved that it hadn't spread.

"So then they said that there was really no reason for me to have a mastectomy, but they wanted me to go meet with a radiologist [radiation oncologist] at Mercy Hospital Cancer Center. They all communicate back and forth very well. So then, in a couple of weeks, I started radiation. I think it was 32 treatments. Radiation was awful. For some people, I know it's not, but my skin burned very, very badly, and I was extremely uncomfortable, and I was extremely tired. I worked half-days through about half of it, but then it got to where I couldn't focus … I got to where I couldn't work at all.

"It seemed like it took me a long time to get over that, but maybe that was because I was so impatient, and I wanted to get back to having the energy to do normal things. I'd always been a person who felt very much in control, active, goal-directed, accomplishing a lot. It was just frustrating. So I finished radiation the second week of August, and by the first of November, I felt really, really good."

Unfortunately, Jo Ann's return to feeling better was cut short by the results of a magnetic resonance imaging (MRI) that she had the second week of November. "When I had an MRI with my first checkup, they called and said that there was a suspicious area, and they wanted to do a biopsy but couldn't schedule it until another week … So I came back on the Monday before Thanksgiving and had the biopsy. The radiologist who was doing this core biopsy said, 'Oh, you know, the odds are pretty small that this is cancer.'

"My husband went with me the next afternoon for the results. We talked to a nurse practitioner. When I saw that the nurse had brought a mold of a breast, I thought, This isn't good. She's going to show us where something is on that mold. I just thought, Not good." Again, Jo Ann and Pat almost simultaneously looked at each other, raised their eyebrows, nodded, and pursed their lips.

Jo Ann's suspicion was confirmed. Less than six months after completing radiation treatment for her first cancer—treatment with side effects that were far from trivial—Jo Ann was diagnosed with a second cancer. After discussing the options with the surgeon, the radiation oncologist, a plastic surgeon, and, of course, her husband, Jo Ann decided to undergo a bilateral mastectomy and reconstructive surgery. "It's hard enough the first time, and you'd think it would be easier the second time, but it's even harder the second time, because you know too much about what may be coming."

After Jo Ann's surgery, the three men in her family stepped up to help the woman they loved. "Pete cleaned the drainage tubes. He gave me a shower. He washed my hair in the kitchen sink. I wasn't allowed to raise my arms, so my older son did all the laundry. My kids had walkie-talkies. They put a walkie-talkie by me and they had one with them, so anytime I needed something, I'd push on it, and here they'd come running. They all pitched in and did everything.

"I'd been home about two weeks and I couldn't stand it anymore. I said, 'Greg, we're going for a drive. We need to return some dishes to some people [who had brought food]. You can get out and take them in, and I will just tell you where to go.' He had his learner's permit—it's 14 in Iowa—so he put me in the car. He put on my seat belt. He would talk to people at the door and say, 'My mom's in the car.' He was wonderful … My sons followed the lead of their dad. He showed them what families do for someone they love." Jo Ann paused for a few moments. She cleared her throat before continuing.

"I've never stayed home very much. I've always worked, and being home that much was very hard. I couldn't do anything. I really had to be very accepting. If the house was not the way I wanted it—oh, well. I made the decision that I was absolutely not going to complain or gripe about things that really do not matter. But I also looked forward to the time that I could do things for myself again, certainly. It was really hard, but it also gave my family an opportunity to prove that they could help … It was good for my children in many ways. I think they learned some tough things that I don't know if any child should have to learn. It made them more compassionate.

"For this walk, my younger son, who just now has turned 13, had earned some money babysitting. He said, 'Mom, I want to give you some money for your walk.' I said, 'Jason, if you'd like to, that's wonderful, but you don't have to.' He said, 'No, I remember how it felt, and I don't want another kid to have to feel that way.' So it was his own idea. It's been a couple of years now. In his life, it's been an eon, but he still remembers what it felt like." Jo Ann and Pat looked at each other and smiled this time.

———

Until transcribing the conversation with Jo Ann Merfeld, I hadn't realized that, despite the fact that she was reared in Kentucky, went to college in Indiana, and has lived in Iowa for the last 23 years, she had the Minnesotan mannerism of beginning sentences with the word "so." Sometimes "so" was a single syllable but, at other times, it was the typical Minnesotan two-syllabled, prolonged "So-o-o-oooo."

Also, typical of many Minnesotans, Jo Ann was somewhat formal when we first met—not unfriendly, not shy, not skeptical, just formal. This personality trait—which, truth told, I *really, really* like—was more noticeable in Minnesota than anywhere else in the country. For example, when people at the Boston 3-Day recognized my drawl, they acted enthralled that a Texan had traveled such a long way for their event. They asked lots of questions—everything from how I raised the necessary $2,000 per event (my fiancé contributed the total amount), to how I had trained in the Texas heat (in the early morning), to what I was planning to do during the 36 hours that I was at home in San Antonio between events (unpack, do laundry, fix a nice meal, pet my dogs and my birds, shave my legs, canoodle, and repack). People at the New York and Washington, D.C., 3-Day events were, in general, less enthusiastic about a Texan among their ranks—maybe it had something to do with the Texan in the White House—but they still asked a lot of direct questions, some of them with a little sauce. "So whudaya doin' in New Yawk?" and "There isn't a 3-Day in Texas that you could have done?"

In Michigan and Chicago, the same questions arose, but they seemed to flow naturally from two-sided conversations, rather than smacking of an oral examination, albeit a good-natured oral examination. In sharp distinction, Minnesotans were almost comically circumspect about asking any personal questions. When I struck up a conversation with someone other than a Minnesotan, I would be asked, almost immediately, "Where are you from?" or "You're from Texas, right?" In contrast, when talking with a Minnesotan, the conversation would be 10 or 15 minutes along before they ventured, "So-o-o-oooo, you're not from around here."

I always said, "No, I'm from Texas," but had I responded, "No, I'm not," I sensed that they would have retreated to another subject that was less personal.

Minnesotans also had the endearing habit of agreeing with someone or urging the person to continue talking by saying "Yup," "Yup, yup," or even "Yup, yup, yup" when they were warming to the subject. I wasn't the only out-of-stater who noticed this. Another was breast cancer survivor Chloe Deodato, who was walking in the Twin Cities 3-Day to celebrate 20 years of knowing her best friend, who lived in Minneapolis. Chloe had also noticed the reticence about asking personal questions and the frequent use of "so" and "yup."

Like Jo Ann's cancer, Chloe Deodato's small, but invasive, breast cancer was an incidental finding adjacent to a palpable cyst. Chloe was 25 years old and working part-time at a Catholic school as the science lab technician in her hometown of Seattle when she found a mass in her breast. "My mom had always had fibrocystic breasts, and she found lumps and cysts. She would get her cysts aspirated, so I sort of knew what to look for as far as lumps. I'd actually found a lump when I was in graduate school and had it checked out. It turned out to be nothing but, in January 2001, I was poking around, and I found a really large lump. I was feeling really uneasy.

"In early February, I decided, I'm going to get this looked at ... You tend to have that gut feeling that something is wrong. I wasn't sure what it was, but I thought, Okay. Lump in breast; it might be cancer. So I made an appointment with my regular doctor, and he looked at it. He was like, 'This is sort of unusual. You should get a mammogram or an ultrasound.' He scheduled that in mid-February. It turned out that the lump that I found was benign, but there was a little area right next to it that they were concerned about because the margins were irregular. So I had the biopsy done in early March.

"A week after the biopsy, I called the doctor because no one had called me. I thought, I might as well call them and see if something is getting held up somewhere or something. They put the surgeon who had done the biopsy on the line, and he said, 'It's cancer.' He got me an appointment that afternoon and talked about all the possibilities for procedures and stuff. Since I had basically no breast tissue—being so tiny—I was like, 'Just get it out of me. I'm not really that concerned about my appearance. I hardly have any breast tissue at all, so it's not like I'd be missing anything.' So I went for the biopsy. I guess they'd label it technically as a 'partial mastectomy' because I have no breast tissue. It would have been a biopsy for anyone else." Chloe grinned, arched her eyebrows, and shrugged.

Her tumor was 0.7 cm with areas of invasive ductal carcinoma. She also had a sentinel node biopsy, which was negative for metastatic carcinoma. "They said it was slow to medium growth. They said, 'Most likely, everything's out, but since it was invasive, we might as well put you on tamoxifen and do the radiation. Since you are darker-skinned, the radiation probably won't be a major problem,' and it wasn't. I had the basic sunburn but, other than the major fatigue, everything was fine."

The etiology of radiation fatigue remains obscure. Chloe wasn't alone when it came to radiation fatigue. I have read everything about the subject that I could get my eyes on because—not to put too sharp a point on it—radiation treatment knocked the straw out of me. When I asked the radiation oncologist for suggestions, he more or less patted me on the head and smiled. He then shrugged and said, "Well, you might try some Tylenol®." (This patronizing manner was aggravating. In fact, by the time I finished radiation treatment, I despised him.)

It may sound like I'm bragging but, before radiation treatment, I was a major hoss when it came to getting it all done. My friends used to say that, instead of chronic fatigue syndrome, I had chronic energy syndrome; during treatment, I was determined to show my stripes and be a super-patient. No schedulus interruptus for me. Extra rest was for sissies. However, radiation fatigue had something else in mind for me.

Within two weeks of beginning treatment, I felt like I was trying to swim in a vat of molasses; the harder I tried, the more exhausted I became. My treatments were at the end of the day, which allowed me to continue working, but by the time I got home, I wasn't always sure that I could walk from the car to the front door. Even worse, the fatigue did not magically abate when treatment was done.

Chloe's description of her daily schedule while undergoing radiation treatment indicated the gravity of the treatment-associated fatigue: "Since it was only a part-time job, I was only working three hours a day anyway. They really didn't care what time I came in. If I needed to sleep some more, I could, which was great. I knew the teaching schedule, so just as long as I got stuff done before class started, it was great. So after I got back from work, I went to radiation. Then I came home from radiation, had a snack, took a nap for two hours, got up and ate dinner, went back to sleep, woke up, went to work. It pretty much zonked me out for a good six weeks or so. The fatigue didn't go away when radiation [treatment] was finished. It took so long to get over that." She shook her head and exhaled.

"A few months later, in October, I finally got the job that I have now. So it was a full-time job, and it took me maybe six months or so doing that full time before I could actually go all day without being tired. It was probably at that point that I realized, Hey, I'm able to do all the things like I did before. Now, definitely, I feel okay."

For all intents and purposes, Chloe faced breast cancer alone. "My boyfriend broke up with me before the first biopsy. He didn't know how to handle it. We haven't had a decent conversation since my diagnosis. He can't talk to me anymore, which is sad, because we were so close in high school. But, you know, I can't do anything about that. It's really his problem, because whatever I try to do to get the friendship back on track, he's not willing to contribute … After my treatment, we sort of did this off and on thing for two years. Last summer, I finally said, 'Forget it. It's just not working.' So he wasn't much support.

"I got a lot of support from my best friend. We've been best friends since fourth grade. It turns out that she's a lesbian, but that's not really important as far as our friendship is concerned. She moved to Minneapolis the week before I was diagnosed, so she was 1,500 miles away, but we talked on the phone a lot."

When I asked about her family's reaction, Chloe said, "Unfortunately, both my parents' mothers died when they were two or three years old, so they didn't really grow up with a strong family background in that department. They didn't really know how to nurture my brother and me when we were growing up. So I was like barreling through all these treatments, and they were saying, 'What's going on with you?' and I'd tell them. I invited them to come along with me to treatments, but they didn't really want to. They were sort of stand-offish. I was basically going through this alone."

The year after Chloe was diagnosed with breast cancer, her mother's annual mammogram showed an abnormality, which turned out to be ductal carcinoma *in situ* (DCIS). Her mother also had lobular carcinoma *in situ*, so she elected to undergo a bilateral mastectomy. About her mother's treatment decision, Chloe said, "She's said, 'Forget this. I don't want to sit here and wait for another surgery.' She just got rid of them. She was 59 when she had the surgery. She didn't bother with reconstruction. She was small-chested—not as small as me—but she really didn't feel the need for reconstruction. After her treatment was when she started being all motherly and nurturing and stuff ... It's very odd. You're supposed to be nurturing toward your little babies, not to your 26-year-old children. At least they're there for me now, so that's good." Chloe laughed and added, "Maybe if they could tone it down."

Chloe's parents emigrated from the Philippines. Her dad came to Seattle in 1971 and found a job within two days, working on a survey ship for the National Oceanic and Atmospheric Administration. In 1972, he returned to the Philippines and married Chloe's mother, who joined him in Seattle the following year. Chloe was born in 1975 and spent her childhood in Seattle. She described herself as "one of those tortured minority kids growing up ... I was an outsider, because I was in honors classes, and there weren't many minorities in honors classes, and I was lower middle class, so I didn't really have anything to impress people with or anything. I was really, really shy, so I wasn't really sociable.

"I didn't have an ounce of confidence until I got into college. Actually, everyone was sort of surprised that I wanted to go to the University of Washington, because it's such a huge school. They said, 'You're so shy. Why don't you go to a teeny-weeny college where you can develop?' I said, 'I've been with the same group of people—the same group of torturers and annoying people—for the last 12 years. I want to go to a place where I'm completely anonymous—where I can just work on being me and develop whatever skills I have and get good at something without having people there to always put me down and antagonize me. That's why I stayed home and went to UW. Besides, they have a good science program there, and I was sure I wanted to go into science at that point."

Chloe's undergraduate degree was in zoology with a marine biology emphasis. After graduating, she entered a master's program at the University of North Carolina at Wilmington, with the intention of becoming a marine biologist. "I went there and, over the course of my one-and-a-half-year stay, we got direct hits by three hurricanes. Consequently, anything that I would have wanted to study was scraped up and taken away by the hurricanes. I wasn't making any progress, because the organism that I was trying to study grows on docks and pilings, so with the winds and the heavy currents, it was scoured off. My advisor would not let me switch projects and wouldn't understand. He basically kicked me out of the program because of natural disasters. He was a complete jerk but, about that time, things in my family were going crazy.

"My parents were going through major empty-nest syndrome because both my brother and I were out of their house for the first time ever. When I was in undergrad at Seattle, I was living at home, but my brother went to undergrad in Wisconsin. He was going through some pretty rough times, too ... Also, right after my advisor told me that he was taking away the funding for my project, we found out that my brother's godfather—my brother and I and their kids grew up together—was dying of lung cancer. All of those things happened about the same time, so I decided to leave Wilmington and go back to Seattle."

The job that Chloe started after completing radiation treatment was as a research scientist assistant at the University of Washington Genome Center; however, this was not the position she applied for. "I got an interview at UW for the lab helper position, which would mean being a dishwasher, basically. One of the guys who interviewed me totally gave me hell about it. 'You've been to grad school. You've got a BS. Why the hell are you applying for this position?' And so I thought I was toast, right? A couple of weeks later, they called me back for another position—this research scientist assistant position. Apparently, the guy who totally chewed me out was the one that recommended me for the position. I had no idea when I started working there that I would be doing this, but I'm actually project lead in a collaboration with Mary-Claire King to investigate mutations in *BRCA1* and *BRCA2*."

Mary-Claire King is the American Cancer Society Research Professor of Genetics and Medicine at the University of Washington. Among King's many, many awards and honors is the Brinker Award from the Komen Foundation. In 1990, King's lab was the first to prove that there is a fairly straightforward genetic link for susceptibility to breast cancer in some families. The genetic mutations in these families were linked to a region in a gene that was later to be designated as none other than *BRCA1*.

At the time that Chloe was hired, King's lab was involved with a study of high-risk families that don't have known inherited mutations in the *BRCA1* or *BRCA2* genes.

This was how Chloe described the research technique for identifying gene sequences: "Basically, we chop up a person's genome into little bits. Each different little segment is placed into a single bacterium. So now we have around 2.5 million *E. coli* bacteria, each with a different bit of a person's DNA inside of them. Each bacterial cell is called a clone. We break the library of clones into pools of 6,000. We have known places in *BRCA1* and *BRCA2* where the sequence doesn't really change much, so we put PCR primers down on those regions and, by screening these plates full of clones, we can tell which wells have segments of *BRCA1* and *BRCA2*." As she described her research, Chloe became more animated. She was obviously enthusiastic about her work.

Although she had far surpassed my understanding of the technique she was describing, I continued to nod and murmur uh-hums, as if I understood what in the Sam Hill she was talking about. "Then we dilute these pools down until we obtain a single colony of clones containing a segment from *BRCA1* or *BRCA2*. We can pull out clones with segments from these genes and therefore sequence either or both genes for that particular individual."

"Wow," I answered. "That's fascinating. So are you and your mother in the study?"

"Yeah, we're an official mystery family. When I first got the position at UW, I was doing DNA preps for six months. I heard that our lab might start a collaboration with Mary-Claire King and might do some breast cancer stuff. I approached my boss at the time, who was heading up the project, and said, 'I'm a breast cancer survivor, and my mother is a breast cancer survivor. Is there any chance that we could take part in this study as study participants?'

"He said, 'Okay, I'll talk it over with the big boss and Mary-Claire King and see if there are any conflicts of interest or anything.'

"We went in for blood tests and had our exons screened." Maybe Chloe had caught on that I was bewildered by what she was talking about because she said, "Exons are the parts of a gene that contain the coding information to make the gene's protein. Each exon is responsible for only part of the complete protein. Anyway, they found no known mutations in our exons, so they said, 'You guys are officially a "mystery family."'" That's a good thing because they were looking for families with no known mutations in the *BRCA1* or *BRCA2* genes. We became study participants and did all the paperwork and surveys for that. For the project I'm doing, I'm actually in one of my freezers at work." Chloe laughed wryly and added, "One of my cousins on my mom's side died from ovarian cancer at age 36, so there's something there.

"After I'd been working on that for a while, my boss said, 'You've been doing amplified DNA preps for a long time. You want to work on something else?'

"I said, 'Yeah, sure,' and there started my involvement with this fosmid fishing process. My boss ended up taking a job at a different company, and I ended up taking over the *BRCA1* and *BRCA2* study. I'm more or less the only person who really cares about what we're turning out. They know that if I continue to be the head of this project that the data are still going to come through, and it's not going to get stuck anywhere, because I'm going to want to know what it is."

When Chloe isn't chopping genomes or colonizing bacteria or breaking libraries or screening plates or diluting pools or pulling clones or sequencing genes or stashing parts of herself in a freezer, she is salsa dancing. She obviously loves it. In fact, when she was talking about salsa dancing, she was almost as animated as when she was talking about her leading-edge breast cancer research. She said that when she and her brother were children, they performed for cultural festivals in a Filipino dance group. This continued through college, but it wasn't until relatively recently that she became interested in salsa dancing.

"It's Latin dancing, and it's really, really fun. I'm meeting a lot of guys." Chloe giggled and flashed a vaguely mischievous smile. "Salsa class is Monday, and I go salsa dancing Thursday and Saturday nights. I go by myself, but there are like five or six guys who I dance with. It's a whole night's worth of dancing. People tell me that I'm pretty good. I'm almost to the intermediate level in the classes that I'm in, and I dance with a lot of intermediate- and advanced-level dancers. I'm thinking about starting tango classes. I pay like 50 bucks for shoes, but I still get more blisters salsa dancing than I do walking. I haven't gotten a blister walking yet, and I get blisters every single time I go salsa dancing." Laughing, she added, "I stopped buying lunch at work, because that's five dollars, and I'd rather spend that money on salsa dancing."

Although she danced with partners, of course, Chloe was usually alone when she trained for the 3-Day. I asked her what she thought about while she walked, and she said, "Things that have happened. What might come. What I might want to study. At this point in my life, I'm like, 'Give it to me. I can take it.' Whatever comes up, I'll deal with it. I guess that breast cancer recurrence is always in the back of my mind, but right now I'm trying to figure out what makes me tick and what I want to do … I'm thinking maybe after this [the 3-Day] that I might start looking at programs and see if I want to go back to graduate school."

Chloe may have enjoyed meeting guys when she goes salsa dancing, but she wasn't going to have much of a chance to do the same at the Twin Cities 3-Day. The word on the street was that, of the 1,960 walkers, only 16 were men. Despite the small number of men who were walking, during dinner the first night of the event, Nancy Mercurio recited "The Top Ten Reasons for Being a Man at the 3-Day":

10. AOL® for Broadband, Motrin®, and New Balance® give-aways make great last-minute gifts.

9. There are no lines at the shower.

8. You get to learn a woman's name just by looking at her name tag.

7. You're the only one who knows what that sink in the porta-potty is used for.

6. It's okay to talk about breasts for three days.

5. It's okay to whip out Vaseline® in public.

4. No matter how much they want to, the women can't run away (referring to the 3-Day rule of "no running").

3. Your new pick-up lines can be tried out, like "Know any good groin stretches?"

2. It's okay to grab and go.

1. A 100:1 ratio.

As with every 3-Day event, the ratio of women to men was nearer parity among the crew members. One humorous anecdote emerged from a conversation between two of those men: As one was walking past a group of women about 20 yards away, he turned his head and yelled, "So, Barb, don't go thinking you'll be coming to my tent tonight." One of the women in the group shook her head, rolled her eyes, and smiled, but did not answer. Another male crew member, who was walking several paces behind the first, looked toward the group and yelled, "Barb, you can come to my tent." He paused before adding, "Who's Barb?"

The Twin Cities Pit Stops also had their share of uninhibited men. One, dressed as a cheerleader with pink pom-poms on his head, greeted us with, "Hey, Twin Cities, you're walking for your titties. Your feet are swellin', you're walking for your melons." And so forth. This energetic soul was even mentioned during dinner the second night when Nancy Mercurio was reading participants' entries in the contest for "The Top 10 Things Learned at the 3-Day":

10. Glide® is no longer just a verb, but the best $6.99 ever spent.

9. While we may not recognize a face, we can tell exactly who someone is by their butt and their fanny pack.

8. A man with pink pom-poms on his head, leading a cheer about titties, is not something to worry about.

7. Moleskin®. It isn't just road kill anymore.

6. When you go into a porta-potty, don't look down.

5. If you scuff your feet on the gravel and pass gas at the same time, no one knows.

4. Boy Scouts rule. (Three troops were on hand at the Twin Cities 3-Day to help us pitch our tents. When Nancy read this reason, there was a standing ovation.)

3. How to walk in flip-flops at 3 AM without flipping or flopping.

2. A hot shower can be better than sex.

1. Random acts of kindness happen everywhere and are, in fact, common at the 3-Day.

Breaking one of the rules by running (okay, jogging) to get a cold soft drink for a woman who collapsed qualifies, I suppose, as one of those random acts of kindness that are so common at the 3-Day. This is what I did for Carolyn Halliday, 52, when she fainted on Day 1. She had just finished walking the entire distance, but suddenly felt light-headed when she was on her way to retrieve her gear. One of the 3-Day staff members was nearby and helped her to a folding chair, while I ran (okay, jogged) for the soft drink. Carolyn felt better almost immediately, attributing her "sinking spell" to a particularly intense hot flash. I was sympathetic, since hot flashes can, indeed, be withering experiences.

You can skip the following description if you know about hot flashes; otherwise, read on: You'll be at, say, a committee meeting, sitting at a table, listening to some self-important, long-winded chairperson droning on about something that you don't give a flip about. Without warning, you find yourself wearing a wool cap, then a wool turtleneck sweater, then unlined wool trousers, then wool socks. You start to fan yourself as unobtrusively as possible, but it doesn't help because you are now being lowered into a vat of molten paraffin.

You begin to pant, puckering your mouth, ever so slightly, as you exhale. Sweat pops out on your upper lip and your forehead, and ladybugs of sweat crawl down between your breasts (or, if you're like some of us, what's left of your breasts). Some of the other committee members glance curiously at you, which only serves to add wool earmuffs and mittens to your wardrobe. You begin to loosen or remove *any* garments that aren't necessary for modesty's sake: the scarf around your neck; the top button of your blouse; your blazer. (*Dammit,* you're thinking, no wonder they call it a blazer.)

With a twinge of near-panic—after all, you *are* suffocating—you blurt out, "Is it hot in here?" The men and most of the women look around at each other and say, "No, not really." But one dear, dear woman about your age says, "It *is* stuffy in here." She then grabs her committee report and vigorously fans herself. You are so appreciative that you feel like kissing her on the mouth. You resolve to do something nice for her the next chance you get—that is, if you survive this furnace that you're in.

If you are compassionate, you will abide by this rule: If a woman who might be menopausal asks, "Is it hot in here?" you will answer, "Yes, it's hot in here," even if it is so cold that you can see your breath when you speak.

Tamoxifen-induced hot flashes and panicky feelings turned out to be a major inconvenience for Carolyn Halliday. Nine months into adjuvant hormonal treatment, in desperation, she started taking low-dose venlafaxine hydrochloride (Effexor®) to relieve the symptoms. This prescription drug is approved for treatment of depression; however, the therapeutic doses for treatment of depression usually range from 150 to 300 mg/day. Halliday was prescribed a fraction of this but still experienced a marked decrease in the frequency, severity, and duration of hot flashes. Had the symptoms persisted, she was considering discontinuing adjuvant tamoxifen treatment.

Carolyn Halliday was 46 years old when she had two weeks of intermittent bleeding from one of her nipples. A mammogram, an ultrasound, and a ductogram were all negative. The bleeding stopped, but two and a half years later, her nipple started bleeding again. "I had been at a workshop, and on the Friday of the workshop, it starting bleeding again, and it was bleeding a little bit more than it had the first time. I called my doctor's office, and they said, 'Don't worry about it.'

"We had a fire-sale vacation to Aruba departing on Saturday morning, so I got home on Friday and told my husband, 'My breast started bleeding again,' and he said, 'Well, they said not to worry about it, so I guess we'll just go, since we can't get anything done at this point.'

"So we went, and we had to change planes. In the airport, I went into the bathroom, and I looked down. I was wearing a white linen blouse and it was covered with blood, so I had to put a half a roll of toilet paper around my boob and wash out my blouse in the sink. We were traveling with our son, and I didn't want to say anything in front of him because I didn't want to alarm him. He was 15 at the time.

"Anyway, we went; carried on. I didn't say anything but was a bit disturbed about the whole thing. Later, when we were in the hotel room, I was standing in front of the mirror in the bathroom and took my breast out, and it started squirting blood into the sink. I called to my husband, 'Dear, can you come here a minute?'

"So he came in—I'll always remember this, because he's such a laid-back guy—he comes into the bathroom and says, 'Hmmm. That can't be good.'" Carolyn laughed as she described his reaction.

"So I finished the vacation and spent the whole time expressing blood. Every time I went swimming, I expressed blood. It was an astonishing amount of blood. By the time I got home, it wasn't bleeding very much. Again, my doctor was not particularly alarmed. I don't think that they ever quite got it. I think they thought that I was exaggerating. They said, 'Well, we have an opening in four or five days.' I went in and he said, 'It's probably a benign papilloma' [a frond-like growth of epithelium and connective tissue growing inside a milk duct]. They did another ductogram and a sonogram, and the doctor said, 'Are you going anywhere this weekend?'"

She underwent a ductectomy, which is surgical removal of one of the lactiferous (major milk-conveying) ducts with a rim of the surrounding breast tissue. The surgeon found an unusually large, but benign, intraductal papilloma. This explained the bleeding from the nipple; however, the pathologist incidentally found DCIS in the adjacent tissue. The process extended to the margins of the ductectomy tissue.

The surgeon later re-excised the tissue surrounding the previous ductectomy site, but DCIS was still present at three of the six margins. At this point, the surgeon offered Carolyn the choice between another re-excision and a mastectomy.

"The pathology report said that I had multifocal cancer; however, when we went to see the medical oncologist, he said, 'You don't have multifocal cancer.' You know how incredibly nerve-racking it is to try to piece everything together, and you're trying so hard to get information and understand. As near as I could tell, it wasn't multifocal as much as it was connected to the length of the duct, and the duct went all over. So it wasn't really multifocal. There was never any invasion. The surgeon said, 'How do you feel about going through another breast surgery?' and I said, 'I would rather go through another breast surgery and hear that I have no options to keep the breast than to just say, right now, go ahead with the mastectomy.'

"So he went in and took three more chunks of each of the margins, and they were all clean. Breast conservation surgery is very much the pendulum swing in the Twin Cities right now. I don't know how national it is, but they were very much in favor of breast conservation surgery. The oncologist, the radiation oncologist, and the breast surgeon were all saying, 'We'll do radiation. We'll do tamoxifen. We don't see any reason to do a mastectomy.'

"In the middle of all this, when I was trying to decide whether to do a mastectomy or not, I was talking to a plastic surgeon about reconstruction and seeing what that entailed, and talking to women who'd had it and talking to women who hadn't had it. So there was a whole gray period in there. It was before the third surgery that I was really trying to make the decision. That was the hardest part … The husband of a friend—he was some kind of doctor—called me and said, 'Carolyn, just do the mastectomy.' He was trying to be helpful.

"Also, in the middle of this, I saw my gynecologist, whom I'd had the most long-term relationship with, whom I've seen for years, and she said, 'I would get a mastectomy, if I were you.' I saw my internist, who was new in my life, and I really liked him, and he said the same thing, but still, I thought, the oncologist, the radiologist, and the breast surgeon are the people who deal with this all day long, and they're all saying that I don't really need to do this. My husband was like, 'Take them both off. Just don't die.'

"All that was nerve-racking. We were both educated people, and it was still draining to even try to get a handle on what was really up. My husband went to all my appointments with me, and we'd come out of each one and ask each other, 'What was your take?' The doctors, too. They're so used to knowing something, and with each person, it's this whole new world that they have to communicate.

"It was very interesting. When I was in the midst of deciding what to do, I would say that most of the people that I knew, without a doubt, wanted me to get a mastectomy. Everybody was trying to be very careful about what they were saying, so nobody was saying, 'Get a mastectomy,' but I know that that was the tenor of most of my friends—I had this really powerful dream. It was like this thing came to me—whatever it was, a voice from the universe, or whatever—that said, 'You're forgetting that you have *you* as a resource. *You* have the power of healing yourself, so you don't need to do the mastectomy. I thought, Well, okay. That felt really powerful." She looked at me to gauge my reaction before continuing. "On one hand, I'm fairly traditional, but on the other, I'm also open to what's out there on the other hand."

Carolyn is a clinical psychologist and has had a longstanding interest in the mind-body connection and its effect on healing, as well as alternative medicine practices. For instance, she used a guided visualization technique during her adjuvant radiation treatments. "I put myself into a really receptive healing state when I went into the treatment room. I would think, Receive the healing. It was less an image and more the sensation of letting the healing come to me. As I lay on the table, I would think, There are many sources of healing in the universe, and this is one of them. I can receive this, and my body also knows what to do for its own healing ... There's a New Age bookstore across the street from my office where I bought a CD of healing meditation sounds. I would listen to that when I had a break, basically reminding myself that my body knows how to heal.

"It seems there is a pretty solid connection as far as being able to reduce pain. It may not necessarily prolong life, but it can definitely improve quality of life ... There has been some reluctance in the medical community to accept the mind-body connection, because there's a whole spectrum. True, there's lots of bad information intermixed with lots of good information, which is very confusing, but some of the ideas may be valid. In some instances, though, there can be a fine line that is crossed when people twist the concept of the mind-body connection to blame themselves, which really concerns me."

I told Carolyn about an excellent book that discussed this very problem. *The Human Side of Cancer: Living with Hope, Coping with Uncertainty*, by Dr. Jimmie C. Holland, psychiatrist at Memorial Sloan-Kettering Cancer Center in New York City. In her book, Dr. Holland calls this phenomenon "the tyranny of positive thinking." She says:

> *For most patients, cancer is the most difficult and frightening experience they have ever encountered. All this hype claiming that if you don't have a positive attitude and that if you get depressed you are making your tumor grow faster invalidates people's natural and understandable reactions to a threat to their lives. That's what I mean by the tyranny of positive thinking ... A good attitude surely leads to the best and most logical approach to getting cancer successfully treated. But I have also known people with positive attitudes, who sought early diagnosis and treatment, and who simply weren't as fortunate. I have seen patients who had no belief in the mind-body connection and who discounted the importance of their attitude completely, yet they survived ... My view is that if a positive attitude comes naturally to you, fine. Some*

people are optimistic, confident, and outgoing in virtually every situation. Your atti-
tude toward illness reflects your attitude toward life in general and your handling of
day-to-day stresses and hassles.

This last sentence became a fulcrum for me when I was listening to people's stories. In fact, of all my sources, Dr. Holland's book was unequivocally the most insightful. That's not an intentional plug for her book. That's a public expression of gratitude. (An aside: Dr. Holland grew up in Texas, too.)

On Monday morning, as I waited at the Minneapolis-St. Paul Airport to return to San Antonio, I skimmed the September 13, 2004, issue of the *St. Paul Pioneer Press*. The day before, the Minnesota Vikings had beaten the Dallas Cowboys 35-17. The headline on the first page of a special Vikings's sports section was "Showing off: The Vikings lay waste to Dallas' vaunted defense as Daunte Culpepper throws five touchdown passes." Below the headline was a full-page color photo. The caption demonstrated (a little sarcastically, maybe?) some typical Minnesotan reserve: "Vikings linebacker E.J. Henderson, right, taunts Dallas receiver Keyshawn Johnson after an incompletion during the third quarter Sunday at the Metrodome. The Vikings' passing game was more productive than the Cowboys' in Minnesota's 35-17 victory."

Yup, yup, yup.

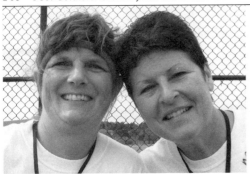
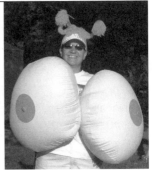

Sisters-in-law Jo Ann Merfeld and Pat Weiss

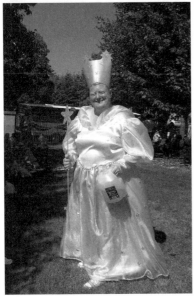
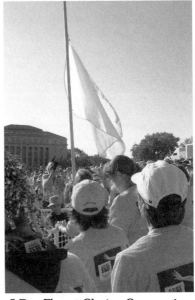

Twin Cities lunch crew volunteer

3-Day Flag at Closing Ceremonies, Twin Cities

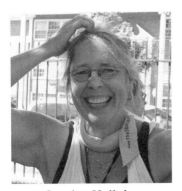
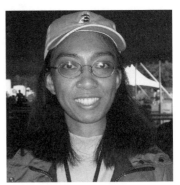

Carolyn Halliday

Chloe Deodato

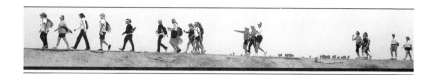

Chapter 7

San Diego
October 1, October 2, and October 3, 2004

Those who lament the "homogenization of the American culture" need only walk 60 miles among Minnesotans and then, a few days later, walk another 60 miles among Californians to discover that significant regional differences persist.

Take, for instance, the justification for honking a car horn. The stoic, blizzard-braving souls of the Twin Cities area are prudent honkers. They must have a sound reason for honking—like urging an elk to move out of the roadway or celebrating a Twins victory in the World Series. A group of people walking beside the road—even if they're wearing feather boas and frilly hats—is not a sound reason.

In contrast, San Diegans are hair-trigger honkers. They honk all the time, at anything, anywhere. When a San Diegan spots a group of walkers—any group of walkers, not just those with feather boas and frilly hats—they honk their horns, roll down their car windows, whoop, and give a thumbs-up. A Minnesotan might nod, but they never, ever whoop or offer a thumbs-up.

What might at first appear to be torpidity on the part of a Minnesotan might instead be a way to conserve energy for the brutal winters. This is only conjecture, of course, but if tenable, it would follow that San Diego's *lack* of brutal winters indirectly contributed to their 3-Day event's bristling energy. Since a San Diegan has no reason to conserve energy for subzero weather, they can squander energy on waving and whooping at 3-Day walkers.

Everything about San Diego was snappy. Cheering stations were noisier. Banners and balloons seemed to be everywhere. A kilted bagpiper, for goodness sake, welcomed us to lunch at Torrey Hills Park on Day 1 by playing, among other tunes, "When the Saints Come Marching In." During lunch at Robb Field on Day 3, a Coast Guard helicopter circled overhead, megaphoning, "Congratulations, walkers." Just before the last Pit Stop on Day 3, a well-coiffed gauntlet of young women from the National Charity League waved fuchsia pom-poms and cheered for us. Even the local media were exuberant.

There were more air horn blasts from 18-wheelers, more full-blast radios in parked cars, more bowls of chocolate candy, more people watching and waving from their front yards and decks, more raised glasses at open air restaurants, more impromptu dancing. More color. More trees. More sunlight. More beautiful young men in Navy whites. More beautiful young surfers in Speedos. More of everything beautiful. There were even more walkers (2,527) and more money raised ($6.7 million) than anywhere else in the country.

The San Diego 3-Day's top honors must have—in Texas cowpoke lingo—done proud Nancy Mercurio, 52, the national spokesperson for the Breast Cancer 3-Day, who calls San Diego home. Nancy grew up in Ventura, north of Los Angeles. She and I are almost the same age, which means that I admired her in the 1960s—if not individually, at least collectively—because she was a California girl. Due in large part to the Beach Boys's exaltation, those of us who weren't wished we all could be California girls.

I still admire Nancy Mercurio. I admire her because she had the *huevos* to answer her destiny. (Wait, wait, *wait*, before you roll your eyes.) I don't use the word casually. In fact, "destiny" is such a lofty concept that, before I even think about it, much less write about it, I brush my teeth and tuck in my t-shirt.

To clarify what I mean by "destiny," let me share a quote from Liz Carpenter, a native Texan and American treasure, who was perhaps best known as press secretary to Lady Bird Johnson. She was the assistant secretary of the U.S. Department of Education during the Carter administration and was dedicating the Frances Perkins Building in Washington, D.C., when she said this: "For many, a single moment occurs in life when history shapes you for a destiny, when you realize your obligations to mankind."

If it was, as I suggest, Nancy Mercurio's destiny to have a crucial role in the Breast Cancer 3-Day, and, if there was, indeed, a single moment, it happened in Liz Carpenter's home state in April 2002. But I'm getting ahead of the story.

Nancy—a certified public accountant (CPA) and marathon runner—walked in her first San Diego Breast Cancer 3-Day in 2001 and was so inspired by the experience that she vowed to walk in all 13 of the 2002 events. Accumulated vacation time and frequent-flyer miles solved some of the logistical problems. Then, to supplement the nearly $25,000 in necessary contributions, she established a Web site and sold t-shirts, hats, and mugs with her coined phrase: "Got Mammogram?" During the walks, she wore a pink jacket that read: "In honor of my mom. 13 cities. 780

miles. 2002 Avon Breast Cancer 3-Day Walks." That jacket figured prominently in the "single moment."

It was at the third event in 2002—the Dallas 3-Day—when event organizers asked her to speak onstage during camp evening activities. Nancy said, "They didn't really know who I was, except that they saw the jacket and knew that I was walking them all. So they said, 'Will you speak in camp tonight about your mom?' and I said, 'Okay.'"

She continued. "At the Dallas walk, people were really grumbling, just whining to the nth degree. 'Shower lines are too long.' 'I'm hot.' So I got up there, shaking like a leaf, and talked about my mom. Then I said, 'You know, the shower lines may be longer than you want them to be, and I know it's hotter than you want it to be, but that's *nothing* compared to waiting for test results when you're a breast cancer patient. That is *nothing* if you're a daughter waiting to give your mom morphine to relieve her pain. That is *nothing*."

The event organizers were so impressed with Nancy's effect on her listeners that they asked her to participate in Opening and Closing Ceremonies for the rest of the 2002 season. The following year, 2003, the NPT [National Philanthropic Trust] and the Susan G. Komen Foundation partnered to continue the 3-Day event and hired her as the 3-Day national spokesperson.

Nancy Mercurio and Howard Sitron, who was then the NPT vice president and chief operating officer of the 3-Day, were some of the most familiar faces at the 2004 events. Participants viewed Nancy on the 3-Day safety video, urging us to adequately hydrate, to stretch hourly while walking, to be polite to others, and to watch where we were going. After the rallying drumbeat of Opening Ceremonies, she also spoke the first words: "We believe." During Opening Ceremonies, Howard congratulated our efforts and made us laugh, but Nancy made us cry, particularly when she narrated the "Survivors' Circle." And it was she who delivered the final, galvanizing words before we started walking on Day 1: "We believe. We believe in a cure. And we will never give up. Until a cure is found, we will never give up."

Howard and Nancy were also largely responsible for creating and sustaining energy and providing humor during evening activities at camp. If their other duties permitted, both of them walked part of the course each day. And, closing the circle, it was Nancy who welcomed walkers and participants into the stage area of Closing Ceremonies, retook the stage in the final minutes, and sent us home with these words: "We believe in a world without breast cancer. And we will keep walking until a cure is found."

Her on-stage persona is so commanding that it may come as a surprise that she was not always comfortable in front of an audience. In fact, the opposite was true. As a high school student in Ventura, California, her parents urged her to participate in Lions Club speech contests.

She said, "I hated it, but I won. It was as if my parents had a vision that I would need it someday. Later, when I got into business, everybody always said, 'You do such a good job on presentations,' but I thought, I hate this. I don't want to do this. If I had the chance, I would always let somebody else do it. I avoided it at all costs."

To fulfill her destiny, she had to first overcome old-fashioned stage fright. Next, she had to make a major decision involving her profession. "At the time, I was working for a medical device company. There were three senior people—the president, vice president of marketing, and me. I was the chief financial officer. I had tons of vacation and frequent-flier miles, so I thought, Let's do it now. I talked to the company president about it, and told him that I was going to participate in all 13 events in 2002, and he said, 'Yeah, that's good.'" Nancy shrugged her shoulders to indicate her former boss's lack of enthusiasm for her cause.

"I was really organized about it. I was flying out on red-eyes. I was in the office as much as I could be. I was doing wire transfers, but the vice president of marketing was having a field day with this. 'Where is she now? What is she doing?' So after the third or fourth walk, or maybe the fifth, one of the employees told me that they had been kind of snippy. The president says to me, 'So how many more of these do you have?'

"I was like, 'Huh?'" Nancy shook her head rapidly, as if trying to recover from being banged on the head, and laughed. "I went out at lunch and got a home equity line of credit—you can do that over lunch now—and I quit. I was making well into six figures, but I was outa there. I decided that I didn't want to work for a company that was so unsupportive. They were in the medical industry. They should have been offering to *sponsor* me for this.

"The company president convinced me to postpone leaving, so I actually ended up staying through the walks, which turned out to be great, because I really did need the money. I flailed for about eight months after leaving the company. I tried to make a go of 'Got Mammogram?' as a business and realized that you have to sell a lot of hats and mugs and t-shirts and pens to make a living—I mean you have to sell a lot of that little stuff."

Despite the obstacles, she persisted, and every time she took the stage, her words were inspiring and emotion-evoking. For many public speakers—barring politicians and some television evangelists—delivering a familiar message with fresh sincerity is challenging, but Nancy said, "It's been a great experience. Could I do it for some other cause? I don't know. For me, you need to have a passion for it. Somebody said that I could do public speaking. I said, 'What would I speak about?' This is a passion, and I don't see myself in the years when this goes away as a speaker ... I get so much energy from the participants—looking out and seeing them." Nancy motioned at a group of walkers who were ahead of us and added, "Knowing what they've done to get here."

She continued. "I think it was a wise decision on the event organiz-ers' parts to have somebody like me be a speaker: a walker who knows what it took to get here and what the expectation is of going home. I'm not sure that you would get that from someone who hadn't participated in the event ... Unless you've walked it, you don't know what the jour-ney has been to get here."

Her passion derives from her experience with her own mother's breast cancer. Nancy's mother, Oneta Deleo, was 61 years old when she was diagnosed with inflammatory breast cancer. "Inflammatory" is a clini-cal term (as opposed to a pathologic term), which means that the lym-phatic channels in the skin of the breast are plugged with breast cancer cells. Fortunately, inflammatory cancer is an unusual clinical presenta-tion but, unfortunately, it indicates that disease is advanced—by defini-tion, at least Stage III. Unlike other types of breast cancer, inflammatory breast cancer does not usually form a distinct mass within the breast tissue; rather, the breast tissue has an ill-defined firmness.

The clinical concept of inflammatory breast cancer got its decep-tively tame-sounding name from its resemblance to an infection: The skin of the breast is reddened, swollen, and warm. And, true to its name, unsuspecting eyes (and fingertips) are sometimes lulled into passing it off as an infection or other benign inflammatory process, at least initially. In fact, lack of responsiveness to antibiotics of a supposed "infection" must always trigger a re-evaluation of these tricky signs and symptoms.

She said, "Mother was a heavier woman and very large-busted—like a 38EEE. She'd have her bras hanging out in the garage to dry, and my brothers and I would say, 'My god, these things are *huge!*'" Nancy laughed and added, "They were kind of like the one I had at camp last night—about that size." (She was referring to an enormous brassiere that she used as a prop during the lost-and-found fashion show the pre-vious evening at camp.)

"I remember I was going up to LA on business, and I checked my messages. My brother had called me to say, 'Mom found a lump on her breast.' It turned out to be inflammatory breast cancer. I think it hit us so hard because we had been through two quadruple bypasses with Dad, and we always thought it would be Dad who passed away first, but, all of a sudden, it was Mom.

"She first went to an oncologist whom several of her friends had used, and whom she had a lot of respect for. He turned out to be a very good oncologist, but I convinced her to go for a second opinion. I took her down to Scripps [The Scripps Research Institute in La Jolla] because some friends of mine had recommended an oncologist from down there. I'm sorry, but I don't remember his name ... Mom told her oncologist in Ventura that she was going to get a second opinion. He was sort of taken aback and asked her, 'Where are you going?' and she said, 'I'm going to Scripps, and I'm going to this doctor.' He kind of perked up and said, 'I'm going to a breast cancer symposium next week, and he's the keynote speaker.'" Nancy chuckled at this, obviously glad that she had been able to take her mother to a well-respected oncologist for a second opinion.

"I ran down all the reports and took her to Scripps. The oncologist there looked at her, and the two doctors got together and came up with a protocol for her. She had chemo first—very aggressive chemotherapy to shrink the tumor before they did surgery ... They were going to remove just one breast, and she said, 'What am I going to do with this?'" Nancy pointed to her own chest and laughed. "'There's no prosthesis that's going to match *this*.' So she fought her doctor on that and got insurance to cover a bilateral mastectomy. No reconstructive. Never wanted reconstructive ... After the surgery, she had chemo again.

"My mom did really well on chemo the first time—lost her hair and got mouth sores, but not really much neuropathy. The side where the tumor was had lymph node involvement. Her prognosis was about six months, but they didn't tell us that at the time. She did pretty well, though, and went into remission." Nancy nodded her head and smiled, obviously pleased that her mother had beaten some bad odds.

She continued. "A couple of years later, my mom said, 'I'm driving along the road, and I'm having these really weird smells. It's like my sense of smell is off.' I said, 'Mom, you need to go to the doctor. When one of your senses goes, it could be a brain tumor. Please, go to the doctor.' She went to the doctor and, of course, she's got a *brain tumor*, which was not anywhere near the site in the brain that controls the sense of smell ... They went in, expecting metastatic breast cancer, right? But it's a meningioma [a benign tumor of the membrane covering of the brain]. Bless her heart, she just sailed along, though.

"Then my dad died of a heart attack in 1997. They had been married for 49 years, and she came out of remission soon after he died. She had been in remission for nine years and had been declared cancer-free. Although she had a great support network—they'd lived in the same community for 40 years—I think something like that can trigger a health issue, which, in her case, I really think it did.

"After he died, she was really funny. They were secure financially, so she started fixing up the house—electric garage door opener, steps up the driveway, automatic sprinkler system. She said, 'I am going to be living in this house, so I'm going to fix it up.'" Nancy laughed, obviously relishing the memory. "My dad was a real homebody, so after he died she started traveling with her friends. She played bridge. She said to me once, 'I always wished that you would meet some nice guy, but I can really see why you like your life being single.'" (Nancy married soon after she finished college but has been divorced for over 20 years.)

She laughed again and continued. "Mom said, 'Now, Nancy, don't get me wrong. I loved your dad, but now if I want to have cereal for dinner, I just have cereal for dinner.' My older brother Tony lived in the same town as Mom, and he started trying to offer lots of advice. I was so proud of her when she said, 'Tony, I buried a husband. I don't need another one.'"

Such an attitude would almost seem out of character for a woman—a woman whom Nancy likened to June Cleaver, as far as being the pluperfect 1950s wife and mother—until her upbringing is considered. Nancy said, "My mom came from an environment where my grandmother was a flapper. She got pregnant with my mom when she was 18. She wasn't married." Chuckling, she added, "My mom always told me, 'You're more her daughter than you are mine.' My grandmother was the most independent woman. She married my grandfather, but when my mom was six months old, he left. Until my mom was in high school there was no contact, no support, no nothing, but then he showed up with a wife and four kids to re-enter her life, and, by this time, my mom had a stepfather and a stepbrother. My grandmother's second husband died of cancer, and she stayed single. I was in kindergarten, so she must have been in her 50s, and she lived into her 80s. She never remarried. She stayed single until she died at 83. She said, 'Nope, I'm not going to have one of those again. Nope. I had one bad one and buried another.' She just loved life. She loved to talk to people. She was not judgmental. An amazing person."

Within a year of her husband's death—and after being in clinical remission for nine years—Nancy's mother was found to have metastatic carcinoma in her liver. At Oneta Deleo's primary diagnosis in 1990, the average survival for patients with inflammatory breast cancer was only about 18 months and, if lymph node metastases were present, the prognosis was even poorer. Obviously, her response to the original treatment regimen of Adriamycin® and Cytoxan® had been remarkable. When she had recurrent disease in her liver, though, she was not immediately treated with the same chemotherapeutic agents that had worked so well the first time around because she had already received the "maximum allowable" dose of Adriamycin®.

A major drawback to high-dose Adriamycin® treatment is the risk of cardiac toxicity (impaired heart function, which may result in fatal congestive heart failure). The likelihood of this side effect increases as the cumulative dose increases. For this reason, Mrs. Deleo was started on paclitaxel (Taxol®). Nancy said, "It was absolutely poisonous to her. She'd done really well on Adriamycin®, but Taxol® just wiped her out … She developed neuropathy and was immediately admitted to the isolation unit. Then they tried a couple of other things. She went for about a year in and out of the hospital before they put her back on Adriamycin®, and she did well again. They were concerned about her heart, but she said, 'Well, *hello.* I'm going to die of something!'" Nancy slapped her forehead with the palm of her head.

"It was at Thanksgiving when she got pneumonia, and she couldn't bounce back from it ... I never resented her weight at all. I was never embarrassed by her weight, because she always took such pride in her appearance, but it was really hard when she got sick. I was her caregiver, but we brought in nursing care because I couldn't lift her. I think that if we had been able to get her back up ..." Nancy's voice trailed off.

"They had put her on Herceptin®, and she was responding, but when somebody gets pneumonia, you've got to get them up. After she got pneumonia, they said no more chemo. By not having chemo, though, her hope was taken away. I told that to her doctor when he said that he was shocked at how quickly she died. I told him, 'Dr. R., you took away her hope. You don't understand how she worked. As long as there was hope, she was going to fight. By not having chemo, her hope was gone.'

"Up until Thanksgiving, she was driving herself to her bridge club and going to parties. So it was around five weeks ... That was the toughest thing I've ever done in my life. I told my brothers, 'If I ever become like that, pay a stranger.' I know my mom was of the era that your kids take care of you. My brothers had no clue. Afterwards, I said, 'I'm having a hard time remembering Mom not sick,' and they said, 'But she looked so *good*.'

"I was slitting nightgowns, putting brand new nightgowns on her, brushing her hair. They'd come into the room and say, 'Doesn't she look nice?' I never told them, 'You missed the diapering part. You missed the skin breaking down.' I never told them, because there was no need to tell them that.

"I really monitored her in-home health care person. These people can be godsends, but they can also be pieces of work. You can understand how some sick people can be bilked of money and taken advantage of. For instance, one woman whom we hired really bonded with my older brother. She thought he was the best thing since sliced bread. My brother called one day and said, 'Mom's buying Mary [not her real name] a condo.'

"I said, '*What?*'

"'She told me that Mom's buying her a condo.'

"I said, 'First off, Tony, I have the checkbook. Second off, I have the durable power of attorney. There's not going to be any condo-buying going on here, so you can just put that to rest.'" Nancy laughed and shook her head.

"I didn't leave Mom at the end. I just took time off from work. I just wanted her comfortable. She was crying and saying that she was ready. You know, she had a priest come in. She wanted a priest. She wanted last rites. I wanted her comfortable. I felt like I'd had more time with her. She never was on that much morphine—we never upped it very much—but five days before she died—it was Christmas Day—we brought in hospice. I had a lot of problems with it afterwards, because I felt a little bit like—I don't know."

She paused, as if searching for the right words. "I wish they had somehow counseled me a little bit more on giving a loved one morphine. We had some problems afterwards, definitely, as a family, but I think she was ready. She'd have really clear moments, and then she'd have loopy moments. We tried not to laugh."

Nancy described the day that she and her nephew brought her mother home from the hospital. "We put her in the living room because it had an ocean view. It was sort of this daiquiri color—we used to call it the 'daiquiri room.' You have to understand that Mom was an interior decorator, so my nephew and I went out and bought linens to match. I bought a cabinet for all the medical supplies, because the home health person had Depends® scattered all over the place." Nancy frowned and shook her head. "Give her her dignity! Her friends are coming to say good-bye. She doesn't want her friends to know she's in Depends®. So we had her all set up. Her Christmas tree was in the corner. We always had two Christmas trees, because my mom wanted one with her Waterford ornaments, and we wanted the family tree, so we always had two.

"My aunt calls, and I say, 'Mom, Aunt Wanda's on the phone. Do you want to talk to her?' Mom said, 'Okay.' I gave her the phone, and she said, 'Wanda, they took me to this convalescent hospital. It's wonderful. First they take you up an elevator.' My parents' house had a steep driveway, so I guess that was the ambulance guy bringing her up the driveway. 'And *then* they bring all your things in.'"

Nancy laughed again, shaking her head, but then abruptly became somber. "Then she kept hanging on and hanging on. She just wasn't letting go. The hospice nurse was coming in every day and saying, 'I'm so surprised to see your mom here.' She finally asked, 'Is she holding on for something?'

"I said, 'Yeah, my older brother. She's holding on for him. My older brother has always been her baby.'

"The hospice nurse said, 'Get him over here.'

"So I called him and said, 'Tony, you need to come over, and you need to tell her it's okay to go.'" Nancy began to cry, but continued, almost whispering. "And he did. He came over that night, and she died in the middle of the night." I squeezed Nancy's arm, and we walked for a while without talking.

She cleared her throat before speaking again. "I slept in the living room with her, and once I fell asleep, and I woke up, and she had died." Nancy paused again, and added quietly, "It was the most peaceful thing, Deb. I think everyone should see death. All the rigidity about her face, the strain—it was all gone. She was back to her ..." Nancy's voice trailed off, then regaining her stage persona, she laughed and said, "Of course, the guys at the mortuary made her look like … 'That's not my mother. Who the hell? What are you guys *doing*? Why did you *do* this?'"

Later, Nancy allowed herself to become reflective again. "I went through a real sorting out period when my mom died. I felt like I had always been available for so many people, but after my mom died, I was surprised at how some of those people were not there for me when, over the years, I'd been there for their autistic child, for instance, and for this and for that. One friend even commented, 'Well, you knew she was going to die.' It just floored me. It was like the lights came on. You really do find out who your friends are … It's a pretty good measure of friendship when you're going through something bad. Friends don't have to really do much—just pick up the phone and ask how you are and what's going on. But those that were there for me …" Nancy paused and nodded. "They were my true friends and still are.

"Until both my parents died, I had never really thought about my life and what I had accomplished. I had never really mourned the fact that I didn't have a family of my own, because I had had other great life experiences: I had friends; I had traveled; I ran marathons; I had been a CPA and worked with a national CPA firm, but then, all of a sudden, my world kind of collapsed." Nancy pressed her lips together and shook her head.

"Going forward as a family, my brothers and I had some real challenges. Even though my brothers had their own families, our parents were the grounding point for the whole family, and that got pulled apart somewhat, at least initially … We struggled so hard for the first couple of years, especially during holidays. My brothers thought that the holidays would be just exactly the same as before, only without our parents. Now, though, we've sort of settled in, figured out what works, but in a different way. We had to recreate the family unit. Her death didn't ultimately pull us apart, which was good, because that was a promise we had made to her—that we would all stay very close—but our dynamics have changed.

"I always tell people that I love the end of [the movie] *Mrs. Doubtfire* when Robin Williams says that your family can be anybody. I love that. I remember the line. I just love that line, because I've always had wonderful friends, and now I look to them. On holidays, sometimes, it won't be all of us getting together. My brothers will go with their families, and I'll go with friends. It took me a long time to realize that that's okay, because it's not my kids, and it's not my family, but it's still a community of people that I can be with, and that's okay to do that."

Like the word "destiny," the word "hope" should not be treated casually; however, unlike "destiny"—a word whose significance can be diluted with overuse—the more that "hope" is discussed, the more gravity it assumes. In fact, most people, including my fiancé—medical oncologist, Tom Fisher, M.D.—are convinced that hope is a pivotal part of the cancer experience. So it was in the story that Tiffany Weis shared with me.

Because her training partners were unable to participate, Tiffany, 35, was walking by herself at the 3-Day. She looked like the type of California girl who inspired Beach Boys's songs, except she looked sad. I struck up a conversation by asking her if she knew the name of the trees that were so common in the area. (I am an amateur naturalist, and when I travel, I try to learn a little about the native plants, animals, and rocks. I'm also nerdy enough to ask complete strangers about stuff like that.) Tiffany told me that they were eucalyptus trees. She seemed to cheer up as we chatted, so I asked her why she was participating.

She said that she was walking in honor of her mother-in-law, who was a cancer survivor, which caused me to quip something tacky about my deceased mother-in-law. I immediately recanted and added that I wished my mother-in-law and I had gotten along better, but that it was now too late. Tiffany then told me that she was also walking in memory of a friend who died from breast cancer in 1996.

Tiffany was 14 years old when she met Judy Henry, an English teacher at the high school that she attended. Tiffany said, "She was a very popular teacher, because she was extremely beautiful, and also because she was younger—only 30-something when we were in school—and was pretty hip. Like, she would say, 'If you're going to ditch, I don't want you to come back to school with a note from your parents lying to me. Just tell me that you didn't want to come to class, and we'll talk about what you don't like about class.'"

In her sophomore year, Tiffany was a student in Ms. Henry's college vocabulary class and described the first day. "I was very social, and walked in and sat down and was yap, yap, yapping to everyone around me. I remember her saying, 'All right, Miss Convivial,' and that was my name forever." Later, she babysat for Ms. Henry's young son, and despite the 16-year age difference between the two women, they became close friends. They had so much in common that they joked that they must have been sisters who were separated at birth. They even had similar physical characteristics: blonde, lightly freckled, slender, and athletic.

"It's funny, but I was so much more like her from the very moment that I met her than I've ever been like my mom. My mom never really taught me how to be a lady, but Judy taught me how to take a bubble bath and how to take care of myself ... I had so much respect for her as a woman. I have to laugh when I'm here—seeing all these women in all these get-ups—because that would be her. She was tough and outspoken and independent and strong, but she'd have had no problem wearing a pink frilly hat."

After high school graduation, Tiffany attended San Diego State and worked at Ralph's (a grocery store), but remained close friends with her former teacher. They went to the movies together nearly every week and even developed their own Christmas tradition. "We would get in the car and drive around and look at Christmas lights for hours. We would go back to her house and have a vodka cranberry. Just one. She loved it because the vodka was in a crystal decanter. She didn't usually keep it there, but she would pour it into the decanter just because she loved the sound the stopper made when she returned it to the decanter—how the crystal sounded, that ding."

Judy Henry's appreciation for sensual details was one of the many things that Tiffany admired about her. "She truly appreciated all the little things in life, always. She was just one of those people who had a lot of energy and a great outlook on life. You hear this about so many people who have passed away, but she just had a zest for life that was beyond anyone else I've ever known. Ten years later, I've never met anyone like her ... She would find beauty and good in everything. I don't understand why those are the people who have to die. I don't get that."

Judy Henry was diagnosed with breast cancer at age 31, while Tiffany was still in high school. After a modified radical mastectomy and chemotherapy, she was disease-free for six years before developing wide-spread metastatic disease. Tiffany said, "I was supposed to come to her English class for a little party—it may have been Halloween—and teach her class the Electric Slide. Remember the dance that all those walkers were doing today at lunch? That's the Electric Slide. She called me that morning and said, 'I have to cancel because I'm not going into school today. My hip is hurting. I might have done something during Jazzercise.'

"I said, 'Okay, we'll just do it another time.' The next week she cancelled because she had a cold that wouldn't go away. They told her she had pleurisy, but about a month later, she still had pleurisy. I said—my mom works for a doctor—I said, 'You need to go to the doctor.' Neither of us was thinking, six years later, that this had anything to do with her prior breast cancer. She had her lungs x-rayed and picked up the films from her doctor, and took them to a friend of my mom's for him to look at. It was full-blown metastatic cancer in her lungs and bone. There was cancer in her sacrum. I was there when the radiologist called back. When he said, 'We found it in your bones,' I went home and got all my stuff and moved in with her and her son, Jason.

"My mom said, 'What are you doing?'

"I said, 'I don't know, but I don't care.'

"I never paused, because it didn't matter. Finishing college at that point just didn't matter ... She had no family. Her parents were deceased, and she had no siblings. I said, 'I'm going to live here,' not knowing how long it would be, obviously. Her son, Jason—I had known her since he was about five—was now a freshman in high school. He's an only child, so I just took care of both of them ... I wanted Jason to have the opportunity to have the rest of his life and to not be destroyed by this experience ... My sister was two years older than Jason, so she took him under her wing with all her friends. Jason is now 28. He was in my wedding and in all of my sisters' weddings. He's our adopted brother. He even looks like us.

"It was shortly after I moved in that she found out that it was in her liver as well. They gave her six months to live, and she lived for three years, almost four with no chemo, just alternative medicine. But she did everything you could imagine. She drank tea; she did these special herbs; she took shark cartilage ... She chose not to do chemo because she had already done it. Had it come back in her other breast or her lymph nodes, she probably would have, but given that it was so severe and that they had told her that it probably wasn't going to help, she decided she wanted to look like herself, and she did. She was very beautiful. She kind of looked like Linda Evans on [the television show] *Dynasty*."

Tiffany's friend was not alone when she turned to unproven treatments for her recurrent breast cancer. In a 1992 article, authors I.J. Lerner and B.J. Kennedy reported that a 1987 American Cancer Society telephone survey determined that 9% of cancer patients used questionable treatments, which are defined as showing no benefit after clinical scientific and/or clinical evaluation.

Tiffany continued. "A lot of her friends were angry. A lot of her friends wouldn't speak to her because they wanted her to go the traditional route, but in her mind—mets in the liver, bone, lung—there was nothing that traditional medicine could do for her. Instead, she went down to a hospital in Santa Monica in Mexico, which I believe helped her a lot, as opposed to some of the other things she did. At the hospital in Santa Monica, they did weird things. For instance, she swam in pools of hydrogen peroxide to get more oxygen to her body." ("Hyperoxygenation" therapies—including hydrogen peroxide baths—are based on the claim that cancer is caused by the lack of oxygen and can be cured if you drown the cancer cells in oxygen. There is no scientific basis for this claim.)

"It was in the days before we knew that hydrogenated oils weren't good for us. These doctors in Mexico were telling her to stay away from hydrogenated oils because it would break down the barrier to your cells. She was in so much pain that she could hardly walk by the time she went down there, but when she came home, she was walking.

"At one point, she tried shark cartilage, but you have to remember that shark cartilage was illegal to bring back across the border from Mexico—like bringing back medicine from Canada now. She was down there at the hospital, and I went to see her. I was going to bring back the supply, and she was going to be coming home in three days. I didn't want her in the car when I brought it back, because she looked sick. All the paperwork that we would have from the hospital—the border officials would know for sure ... I can remember making it back across the border and pulling over at the very first place there was a gas station, and

I just threw up ... I went back other times by myself. I didn't want to go myself, but there was nobody else to go with me, and I swear my mom never knew about it.

Shark cartilage was another alternative treatment for cancer, whose alleged value was based on laboratory experiments showing that direct application of shark cartilage retards the growth of new blood vessels. Since new blood vessels are needed in order for cancer to grow, the reasoning was that eating powdered shark cartilage would slow tumor progression. The problem with this idea was that if a person swallows a protein—any protein, including shark cartilage—it is digested and eventually broken down into its constituent amino acids. It is certainly not absorbed into the bloodstream as a big, gnarly protein.

"I'm from a small beach town. I had driven places, but certainly never across the border. There are no rules when you're driving in Tijuana. You don't know which direction to go, and everything goes in circles. It's horrible, and if you do something illegal, you're going to be pulled over because they love to pull Americans over. At the time, it was really bad. There was a rash of young kids from this area going down there to drink, because you only have to be 18. They were just getting drunk, making a ruckus, causing trouble ... I remember thinking that if they want to arrest me, then they can, because my friend is going to die, and if this is what she believes is going to make her better, to give her the hope and the inspiration to get her through another day—well, they can arrest me.

"I didn't know if shark cartilage was going to do anything. I really didn't care. It was more about what it was doing for her mental well-being. I truly believe that I saw a transformation in her every time she thought that something was going to work ... I told my friends, 'If this is what she believes will make her better, I'm doing it. What else does she have? She has nothing else.' She needed a foundation to start from to get better—to want to get better ... Of course, some of the things that she did were clearly of no benefit to her.

"There was a group of doctors here in downtown San Diego, and I would take her to their office. The waiting room would be crowded with people. I remember these farmers from Illinois or somewhere. They had no money. A mom and a dad and their daughter, who was about 14. The daughter obviously had some kind of abdominal cancer. Her stomach was distended out to here. These people had mortgaged their farm to give their daughter some hope. Those doctors ended up being arrested. One of them was on the run. It was all a big hoax." She shook her head disgustedly and exhaled audibly. "Thank goodness, Judy died before she knew this part.

"Still, as sick as she was, there were certain things that she would do—like Essiac® tea that she would boil all day with all these crazy herbs—that would help her mentally, and her mind would help her body, because she believed they would." (Essiac® tea is based on an herbal remedy containing burdock, Indian rhubarb, sorrel, and slippery elm. It was developed and marketed by a Canadian nurse. Both prospective animal studies and retrospective human studies have shown no antitumor activity.)

Tiffany nodded emphatically as she continued. "The mind-body connection—I'm telling you—I saw it. Two years into her disease, she clearly should have been a lot worse off. It was a combination of the tea and something else that she was drinking. It was amazing. She wanted to go on walks. The energy she had was just phenomenal. She had all her color back. She wasn't getting sick all the time. It didn't last for only a week or a month, but for a few months."

Despite temporary improvement, Judy's condition eventually began to deteriorate. Tiffany said, "When she was sick, she was very angry. The message I tried to give her was that whatever else you might believe in—God, Buddha, any religion, it doesn't matter—you have to believe that there's something better. You have to believe that, or you're not going to have any peace ... For a year, she struggled with the idea that if there were someone good taking care of us that this wouldn't be happening to her. She finally decided that she was going to read the Bible, and when she died, there was the Bible next to her. In it, she had highlighted a verse. I don't remember the verse, but it indicated that she finally got it, and I think she was ready to go.

"She had spells of anxiety when she wanted out of her skin. She was in pain and moaning. She was very scared of dying and never wanted to be alone. I slept in her bed every night, and we held hands. At the end, though, I think that verse in the Bible had finally taken the fear out of it for her."

Tiffany seemed a little apologetic when she described lying in bed with Judy—as if such intimacy might be misinterpreted—so I told her the story about lying in bed beside my father when he was near death.

As I mentioned in the Introduction and elsewhere, my father was diagnosed with a highly aggressive brain tumor in June 1997. He underwent three craniotomies (brain surgeries) over the course of 11 months. The first two operations resulted in minimal cognitive and motor deficit. (In fact, one of our family's half-jokes was that we weren't sure what he'd been doing with his brain all these years since removing chunks didn't seem to affect him.) The third operation, however, silenced all our gentle ribbings. He was bedridden until he died four months later.

After his last surgery, I drove from San Antonio to Austin, where he and my mother lived, nearly every Saturday afternoon for an overnight visit. I did this to give my mother and cousin a little break. I also did this so that I could spend some time with my dying father.

One Sunday morning, I awoke from where I had been sleeping on the couch in the family room beside my dad's rented hospital bed. I watched and listened as he struggled to rouse himself. I use the word "sleep" for simplicity's sake. Toward the end, on morphine and with the tumor clawing its way through his brain, he was increasingly somnolent, drifting in and out of semiwakefulness.

When he finally mumbled, I went to his side and squeezed his right hand—the one that still had a bit of movement and sensation. He squeezed back and said my name. I let down the side rail, and for the first time in maybe 35 years, I lay down beside my father and put my head on his chest. I felt his right arm wiggle slightly at my side. I thought I might be hurting him, so I moved away some to free his arm. Shakily and slowly, he raised his arm and put it around my shoulder, patting me and saying, "I love you, Deb."

I responded in kind. He tried to tell me something, but despite listening as carefully as I could, and urging him to repeat himself, I could never be made to understand what he was trying to tell me. I finally said, "Daddy, I'm so sorry, but I can't understand you."

He answered, remarkably clearly, "I can't understand you either, Deb."

I smiled at this dear man and said, "It seems we spend our whole lives trying to understand each other, huh, Dad?"

He paused, as if searching for words, and answered, "I guess so."

We lay still for a while, my head against his chest. I listened to his shallow, ragged breathing, which was occasionally interrupted by a soggy-sounding cough. Then I softly sang a few old Baptist hymns, including his favorite come-to-Jesus-hymn, "Just Am I Am." At the end of each, he whispered, "Good."

There we were, two people who loved each other deeply, but who continued, in the literal sense anyway, to have trouble understanding one another. Still, though, as I lay there, I was peaceful. In spite of knowing that I would soon lose this man who had been not only a father but also a mentor, a medical colleague, and a best friend, I was still peaceful. My father seemed peaceful, too. He—as does every other creature on this planet—deserved that near the end.

Despite her dismal prognosis, Judy survived long enough to see her son graduate from high school. Tiffany said, "She just kept saying to herself, 'One more day, just one more day.' She just had to see her son graduate at the high school where she had taught, and she did. I wheeled her into the auditorium in a wheelchair. She was so sick. She was so proud, though, to be there. She fought so hard to be there that day that it was almost like it was time to let go. She didn't die until the following January 21.

"It was almost like one of those stories you see on TV—you don't think it really happens—when a community comes together. It got to the point where she was taking off too much time, and she used up all of her disability and sick time. I had written some letters and the whole community came together. All of the teachers throughout the entire district pooled their sick days so that she had an additional year off with pay. The district said no, but we fought it, and she won. A lot of the teachers who pooled their sick days were there at Jason's graduation. They may or may not have known it, but they helped her make it to Jason's graduation."

Tiffany was at Judy's bedside when she died. "We had moved her into the hospital for the last two weeks. Her body had kind of quit, and they said that she was in a coma, but I don't think she was in a technical coma. I think it was that she couldn't get her brain to make her lips move. I was there for nine hours that day. I was talking to her and telling her to just let go. 'You can't fight anymore. It's going to be okay. I'll take care of Jason.' Tears were streaming down her face. There were other people there that saw it. I was so glad that I was there, because she had always been very afraid of being alone ... Her son wasn't there. I had called and said, 'You know, I don't think things are going so well,' and he said, 'Okay, that's fine.'"

Tiffany continued. "You know, Jason had said good-bye so many times already—when we thought it was the end but then the next morning she would be fine ... She went into the hospital this one time, and I thought that that was it. I went home to her son and was really trying to prepare myself because I really didn't think I was going to see her the next morning, but she called and was perfectly fine."

Tiffany put her fingers on her temples, bowed her head, and slowly shook it. "It was like this roller coaster of waiting. It was such a weird psychological game. Your mind would be wanting, in some sense, relief for her, relief for you, but then she'd be okay, and I'd think, Thank God. Still, I knew that she wasn't really okay, so then there'd be like this almost ..." She paused, obviously striving for emotional honesty, and then continued. "Not resentment—I never felt resentment—but I'd almost feel a little angry, because I thought, I can't do this again, but I did. I didn't do it because I had to. I did it because I wanted to.

"I really always felt like something magical was going to happen, and she was going to survive. When I look back, I think it did. She lived for three years, almost four. She saw her son graduate. She had a lot of hope. I've learned from these experiences that you really have to believe. I think there was a time—I know this from nearly dying in childbirth—when I was really mad at God."

Tiffany was referring to a severe complication (placenta increta) that followed the delivery of her daughter. Tiffany lost nearly 3,000 cc of blood within a few minutes, and was, in fact, near death by the time the bleeding was controlled. Her recollection of those moments included the doctor screaming, "We're losing her! We're losing her!" and the overhead speaker in the Labor and Delivery Room blaring, "Code Blue."

She described her emotions after this near-catastrophe. "I consider myself a good person, but I really was angry. I never stopped to look at the fact that I didn't die, and my daughter was healthy, and all those things. Like with Judy, too. My husband once said, 'You never cry about Judy.'

"I said to him, 'I cry all the time inside, but you know what I figured out?'—I don't know how I came up with this—'You know how many people in this world never met her? What a bummer for them. I wanted the rest of my life with her, but I'm so privileged that I had her in my life for as long as I did. Judy and I got to say all the things that really mattered.'"

Tiffany did, however, cry at the San Diego 3-Day. She said, "I am walking in the event by myself, so I ate dinner and took a shower, and I was walking around and stumbled upon that Remembrance Tent. I remembered them saying that there was a certain area that would be set up, but I didn't really pay that much attention. When I walked in, the feeling reminded me so much of Judy. She had developed this huge interest in that stuff before it was really big—Tibetan music, little feng shui fountains. People thought she was crazy or cult-worshiping, but when I walked in that Remembrance Tent, it had that feeling about it. It was very unlike me, but I picked up the pen and I signed that tent to her. It was overwhelming. I wasn't expecting it. I don't cry in front of people— I might get teary-eyed—but I cried as hard as I ever have.

"Breast cancer, no breast cancer, breast cancer survivor, it wouldn't have mattered—Judy would have embraced something like this. She would have walked this 3-Day with me in a heartbeat, if I would have asked her. If she were alive, I'm sure that we would still be side-by-side friends."

———

Nearly everyone leaving the Remembrance Tent appeared to have been crying. Many people also became emotional at a park that we passed through on Day 3 of the San Diego walk. Three miles from Embarcadero Marina Park, which was the site of Closing Ceremonies, the San Diego 3-Day route passed through Spanish Landing Park. Within this park is one of Richard and Annette Bloch's Cancer Survivor Parks. Richard Bloch was a cofounder of H&R Block and a cancer survivor. When he was 52 years old, he developed shoulder pain, which was eventually determined to be secondary to advanced lung cancer. His surgeon told him, "It is inoperable. It is malignant. If I were you, I would get my estate in order." That was in 1978.

Richard and his wife, Annette, were determined that he would survive cancer. One of their first steps was to seek a second opinion. (In their writings, they repeatedly stated that obtaining a second opinion should be mandatory.) And one of the last things they did together (Richard Bloch died of heart failure—not cancer—in July 2004) was to write an article about the importance of a positive attitude when dealing with the diagnosis of cancer. In the intervening 26 years, they touched countless lives through their books and articles, and through the R.A. Bloch Cancer Foundation. They also conceived of Cancer Survivors Parks. Currently, there are 21 such parks nationwide.

Like Richard Bloch, Linda Dreyfuss's symptoms were initially attributed to benign causes, and like Richard Bloch, when Linda Dreyfuss, 54, was correctly diagnosed with Stage IIIc ovarian cancer at age 46, she was told by an oncologist that she had no chance of recovery. Linda said that the oncologist's parting words to her were, "Go home and write your will."

Linda said, "I was so terrified. So absolutely, awfully upset ... The oncologist was probably being realistic, but he was tactless. The diagnosis may be bad, and you can give patients facts, but what angered me—what I resented—was anybody taking away hope. He just slashed any hope ... I was devastated. I cried. I cussed. I was very depressed. Angry as hell. I was so extremely angry. I was most upset about my daughter, and leaving her alone, she being an only child and me being divorced.

"Of course, I called my parents who live in Los Angeles—I live in San Diego—and through their contacts and my brother and sister-in-law, who were involved with a big cancer organization in LA, they found the head of gynecologic oncology at Cedars-Sinai [Medical Center], whom they knew, and who was gracious enough to take me on ... She came in the first day that I met her and said that she had patients who have already survived eight or 10 years. She was a breath of fresh air for me, even though I still knew what the mortality rate was."

The gynecologic oncologist who treated (and restored hope to) Linda Dreyfuss was Beth Young Karlan, M.D., who is director of the Women's Cancer Research Institute, the Division of Gynecologic Oncology in the Department of Obstetrics and Gynecology, and the Gilda Radner Cancer Detection Program at Cedars-Sinai. Dr. Karlan is also professor of obstetrics and gynecology at UCLA School of Medicine.

Linda described Dr. Karlan as being brilliant, but she also talked at length about her appearance. "Dr. Karlan never came into the exam room in a white lab coat. She was always dressed in the nicest suit and accessories. Never, ever have I seen her—except during surgery—in anything but the most beautiful outfits. The only thing she ever did differently during the exam was put on gloves. I looked at her and thought, Omigod, she's like an angel. Very confident. Very sweet. It made all the difference, in comparison with this other guy who said, 'Go home and write your will.'"

Perhaps taking a cue from her beloved doctor, Linda dressed up for all 12 of her chemotherapy treatments. She said, "I would go into treatment dressed as if I were going to work. I dressed in nice clothes. I put on make-up. I always felt crummy coming out—not sick, but tired—but, I thought, I'm going in there with my head held high, looking like a queen. Every single time, I was dressed up to go in to have chemo. Jewelry. Make-up. I had no eyelashes or eyebrows, so I put some on. I always wore my wig. I figured I was going to go in there looking as good as I could, because it made me feel better."

Linda had an excellent clinical response to the first six cycles of combination agent chemotherapy (Carboplatin® and Taxol®). Dr. Karlan told Linda that receiving an additional six cycles of Taxol® was optional. Linda not only wanted the additional treatment but, after completion, she experienced emotions that are surprisingly common among cancer patients. "As much as I wanted to have chemotherapy done, I cried after the last treatment, because I felt like I was being shoved out of a nest, like a little bird. Shoved out and told to fly, and I wasn't ready to do that. By the time I had my last treatment, I was ready for it to be over, but then I didn't want it to be over. I knew the chemotherapy was doing something. My CA 125 plummeted after the first two chemotherapy treatments and had stayed below 5 throughout treatment."

Linda also received tamoxifen for five years and said, "I felt the same way after five years—having to get off tamoxifen. I don't care. Give me a placebo. I just want to know that my CA 125s are going to stay low."

After Linda's third cycle of chemotherapy, Dr. Karlan asked Linda and her family to enter an ongoing study of cancer incidence among Jewish women who were at high risk of ovarian cancer based on family history. Alexander Liede of Toronto was the lead investigator and principal author of the study, which was published in *Journal of Clinical Oncology* in March 2002. Dr. Karlan, Linda's doctor, was the second author.

The study concluded: "The excess risk of breast and ovarian cancer in Jewish women with a family history of ovarian cancer is largely attributable to mutations in *BRCA1*." Unfortunately, the study also concluded: "Intensive surveillance by use of CA 125 and ultrasound does not seem to be an effective means of diagnosing early-stage ovarian cancer in this high-risk cohort."

The tests performed in connection with Drs. Liede and Karlan's study confirmed that Linda's cancer was, indeed, associated with a genetic mutation. Linda said, "I was first tested. I'm a *BRCA1* carrier. Looking at the family tree, they have decided that it was my mom's father who was the carrier. We did find out that three of the four siblings in my family are carriers. My other sister and my brother are carriers. My youngest sister is not. My daughter is a carrier. My mom's two brothers are carriers. My uncle—my mother's older brother—just had a mastectomy three days ago. His son—my first cousin—is a carrier. My mother's other brother has five daughters. One of them died from ovarian cancer at age 43. Of the remaining four sisters, only two have chosen to be tested. One of them is a carrier and one of them is not. Other cousins and even second cousins have been tested, and no one else is a carrier."

Linda's daughter, Shana, was a senior in high school when Linda was diagnosed with ovarian cancer. Although Shana had genetic testing at the same time as her relatives, Linda said, "Shana did not elect to find out the results until three years later. She kind of suspected that she was a carrier, but I think she needed to go through some processing. She needed to be ready to find out her results. She was over 18 when she had the test done, and much as I might have wanted to find out the results, I couldn't. She had to do this on her own, when she was ready. At around 21 or 22, she decided to find out.

"Since finding out that she was positive, she has entered into many voluntary studies for people that are *BRCA1* or *BRCA2* carriers who have not had cancer ... She was in a study at UC San Diego that was mainly about how diet contributes to cancer. She was followed by a nutritionist for maybe a year. That first study connected her to the NIH—National Institutes of Health in Washington, D.C.—for a monitoring study. She wasn't eligible for that study until she was 25. So last January, the NIH flew her out to be tested for two days straight with every test conceivable, base-lining everything. They are committed to doing this for the next 30 years, at least for now—for flying her out, once a year, to track mammograms, CAT scans, PET scans, MRIs, vaginal ultrasounds, blood work, you name it, plus two days worth of interviews with social workers, psychologists, and doctors.

"My daughter has this willingness to do any study presented to her, if she is eligible, not only for her own sake, but because she has this need to help others. I'm just so proud of her for doing this NIH study because not everybody would be willing to go through what is necessary ... I believe that doing this study was partly a cathartic process for her and partly her way of controlling the situation, in addition to being a way to help others. I truly believe that she's trying to grasp at a meager part of control or involvement for herself. It's not a selfish reason at all, but it should be. It's her life. She understands that the knowledge reaped by participating in this study is so valuable. The more you know, the more you can ask questions, and the more you can be proactive about symptoms." Early on, Linda had justification for this approach.

Linda was 21 years old when her own mother was diagnosed with breast cancer. She said, "My mother is a 32-year survivor of breast cancer, so my two sisters and I thought that, if we were going to get any kind of cancer, it was going to be breast cancer. My mother had two mastectomies, 10 years apart. They weren't related cancers, but they were mirror images of each other ... Between the time she had the first one and the second one, my sisters and I would gather on the bed when we were in town together. We had all decided that if we were to get breast cancer, we would do both breasts at the same time ... My dad's sister also died of breast cancer, so we had it on both sides. We didn't dwell on it. We didn't have a lot of information in those days. We knew about my mom, but nobody knew about genetic tendency. You kind of suspected, but there was nothing to really base it on during that period of time.

"I had not a clue that this would *ever* happen to me, even though my younger cousin had had ovarian cancer. I thought that was a fluke. I had no idea." Linda shook her head for emphasis and said, "No *idea*. But, then again, until being genetically tested and going through all of that education, I didn't know that there was a genetic connection and that the predisposition was so great. When I found out, I was devastated—totally, 100% devastated." Linda closed her eyes and shook her head. "I thank God for parents who just took the bull by the horns and ran with it."

Linda's parents and daughter met us along the route and brought along Gold, a Labrador/Golden Retriever mix. Linda's mother and daughter were in clown suits, and Gold was dressed as a bumblebee, complete with cape and bobbling antennae. Gold was beautiful but aloof. When I commented on this, Linda said, "He does not like putting his cape on when we go out in public. He is humiliated. You would see a different demeanor with the cape off, with that bumblebee costume off of him. He is humiliated beyond humiliation. He's a fabulous, fabulous dog, though. Unlike him, the dog I just turned back into the organization in August loved to dress up. Last year on the walk, she was a pink butterfly, and she loved it. Omigod, you put those pink wings on her and her little baubles and her little tutu, and she was in seventh heaven. In fact, when I turned her in at graduation, I painted her toenails pink. She was all girlie. Gold does it, but he doesn't love it. He has no passion. He hates the concept, but he looks so *cute!*" Linda laughed like a proud mother.

The organization that Linda was talking about was Canine Companions for Independence. According to their Web site (www.caninecompanions.org), "Canine Companions for Independence is a non-profit organization that enhances the lives of people with disabilities by providing highly trained assistance dogs and ongoing support to ensure quality partnerships."

Linda became a Volunteer Puppy Raiser near the end of her chemotherapy. She said, "I had maybe one or two treatments left. Shana and I had for a few years been going to the Shakespeare Festival in Ashland, Oregon. We had walked into a theater and sat down a little bit early for this one play, and this family of four walks in with a service dog in training. The two of us, being that we had our own family dog at home, bombarded this family with questions as this seven-month-old dog sat through an entire Shakespearean play—or slept through it. When I got back to San Diego, I found out that my vet was raising one, and learned more about it. Since then, I have raised four Canine Companion puppies in the classroom [Linda is a second-grade teacher], and am due to get my fifth this Wednesday. This was the result of my need to do things now. Before, I'd always write checks for charities, but I knew I had to get involved somewhere. This turned out to be it, and it just fell into my lap. I've been extremely involved with it for the last five years.

"It involves taking the puppy at eight weeks, raising it, going to class *every* other week, and then socializing it out in public in order to practice our commands. I turn the puppy back in at a year and a half, and, at that point, professional trainers work with the puppy. Less than 30% of these puppies make it to being a service dog. If they don't, I have first choice to keep them, so I win either way. Raising the puppies came with my need to start to help others in whatever way—my need to do this because of the family history and Shana and humankind."

Linda also became involved in other volunteer outreach activities, particularly with other women who had been diagnosed with ovarian cancer. She realized that women with ovarian cancer have far fewer well-organized support groups and outreach opportunities than those with breast cancer. She said, "I had no peers at all who had gone through any kind of cancer or any kind of devastating disease like this to look to for support. Knowing the mortality rate of ovarian cancer, I was not about to join a support group, because it's a terminal illness. I didn't want to be brought down any more than I already was, so I didn't go to any kind of support group at all. For breast cancer, there's Reach For Recovery®—people that come to you. I think that would have been helpful, but I did not want to sit in a group of people crying. At that point, I didn't want to hear anybody else's sad story. That may have been selfish on my part, but it was a survival instinct.

"After I finished chemo and got back to work, I decided that I was going to reach out to anybody going through chemo for breast or ovarian cancer, in any way that I could. I wanted to try to help them get through the process, to listen, to answer questions. I wanted people not to feel totally alone through the experience and isolated, like I had felt. Of course, I had family and friends for support, but it wasn't the same as having a peer … If somebody knew somebody that was in my age range that was going through chemo, I gave the friend my name. I said you could tell anybody that wanted any kind of peer support that they can call me, or you can get their number and I will call them. I have talked to people across the country. People that I don't know. People that are friends of friends who are going through either ovarian cancer or breast cancer.

"People say that I do all this stuff for other people. You know what I think?" She shook her head and lowered her voice. "After being hit with a big disease, I do now the things that I had wanted or planned to do in my future. You never know. Nobody knows what tomorrow's going to bring. It's a need I have to do stuff *now*. I think that's where I have this absolute passion to be doing something *now*, to give back *now*."

She paused and then added, "I know the cloud's out there. It's always in the back of my mind. I don't dwell on it anymore because I've gotten to this point, but I know with ovarian cancer, you're never cured. You're in remission, and you can always go out of remission. I think that's what drives me to do what I can. It's just my need to do things now, because if it does catch up to me, I won't be able to."

In October 2004, Linda was nearly eight years out from her diagnosis of advanced ovarian cancer and, for the seventh year in a row, she was walking in long-distance events for breast cancer. She looked absolutely fabulous, dressed in a pink camisole, pink angel wings, and fuzzy, pink-baubled antennae. She was wearing jewelry and make-up—including lipstick, of course—with matching shade fingernail polish. To borrow her phrase: very girlie.

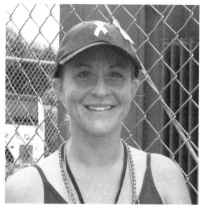
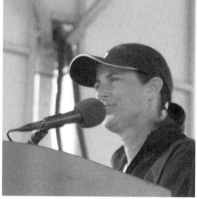

Tiffany Weis   *Nancy Mercurio*

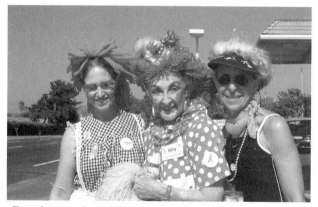

Family members Shana Dreyfuss, Rita Brucker, and Linda Dreyfuss

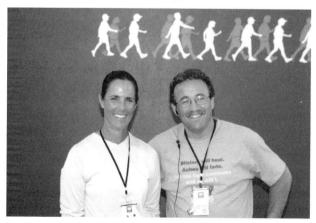

Nancy Mercurio and Howard Sitron

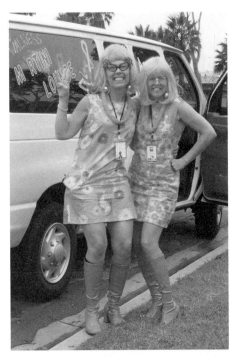

Sweep crew members (and sisters)
Pam Roach and Louise Adams

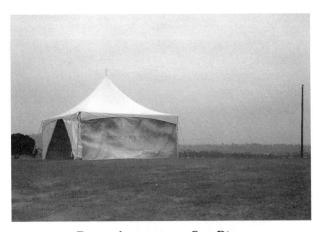

Remembrance tent, San Diego

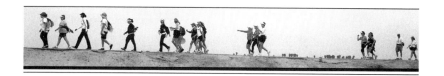

Chapter 8

Los Angeles
October 8, October 9, and October 10, 2004

As I waited to board the plane for Los Angeles on Wednesday, October 6, 2004, Mount St. Helens's recent antics were CNN's lead story. The ruckus had started on September 23, with a swarm of shallow earthquakes. Seismic activity increased to three to four events per minute on September 29, prompting the U.S. Geological Survey to issue a Volcano Advisory (Alert Level 2). On Friday, October 1, Mount St. Helens had what was called a "small explosion," blowing a cloud of smoke and steam. A second eruption on Saturday was followed by 50 minutes of harmonic tremor—an indication that magma might be making its way towards the surface. With this development, the alert level was raised to 3, and thousands of people were evacuated from the mountain, including visitors at the Johnston Ridge Observatory, 5 miles away.

The hazards scientists' predictions were correct. On the following Monday, October 4, the volcano had a 40-minute emission, and on Tuesday morning, John Ritter, writing for *USA Today*, reported a "spectacular burst of steam and ash, towering more than 2 miles high …" In his article, entitled "St. Helens Closer to Big Eruption," Ritter continued:

> *The blast was the biggest yet since Mount St. Helens woke up two weeks ago. The USA's most active volcano seems to be rumbling toward the strong eruption scientists have been expecting for days. Or small daily spews could persist. Or maybe Tuesday was the finale … Scientists say there's more than a 70% chance that Mount St. Helens, which until Friday hadn't erupted in 18 years, will delight its fans with a strong eruption. Few expect it to approach the intensity of 1980, when 1,300 feet of the mountaintop blew away.*

Although my destination that morning was two states away from where Mount St. Helens was delighting its fans, CNN's billowing images and Ritter's rumbling words still gave me pause. I recalled the triangles and lines on the maps that researchers showed us after Mount St. Helens blew in 1980. The triangles, which signified volcanoes, were not only scattered in the Cascade Range, but were also stacked in California's

Long Valley area, and the lines running up and down the California map were the San Andreas fault and its branches, including one tentacle, the Puente Hills fault, under Los Angeles.

I also remembered that around the time St. Helens blew in May 1980, there were some newsworthy earthquakes in the Long Valley area of eastern California. (I later checked on this. There were four magnitude 6 earthquakes.) The crusty exchanges among the West Coast's volcanoes and earthquakes and tectonics are complicated, of course, but if Mount St. Helens were about to blow again, would that mean that California might also be in for some striking and slipping? Was Mount St. Helens signaling that a tectonic plate was fixing to lurch westward and, like a giant spatula, flip California over onto Nevada? Maybe so, but I folded the newspaper, turned my back on the television, and boarded the plane anyway. After all, I thought, you can't live your life in fear of recurrence, whether of a natural disaster or of breast cancer.

In her excellent book, *After Breast Cancer: A Common-Sense Guide to Life After Treatment*, author Hester Hill Schnipper expresses this concept cogently:

> As the months passed and the end of chemotherapy finally arrived, I learned the second important lesson. In retrospect, the crisis of diagnosis and the difficult months of physical treatment are almost the easy part. The real challenge comes with living with breast cancer. It is clear that the goal must be to live as though the cancer will never return. Living any other way, mired in anxiety and sadness, means that the cancer wins, whether it recurs or not.

———

Courtney Lercara-Zinszer was 33 years old when she was first diagnosed with breast cancer. Eight years later, at 41, she said, "In one sense, I feel that I'm scared every day that it's coming back. Every time I get a bruise on my leg or get a headache or I feel disoriented and bang into something, I think, Omigod, it's brain cancer. I must have brain cancer. It must be in my bones. This hurts. That hurts. On the other hand, I think, No, I can't get it again. Not a day goes by that I don't think about it.

"I've lost so much brain power. I don't even know what my IQ is anymore, but it can't be very good. I frequently can't remember things. It's chemo brain." Courtney rapped her forehead with her fist. "When people try to tell me there's no such thing as chemo brain, they're fools. I haven't had chemo in so long, but I'll be talking, and in the middle of the sentence, I'll lose my train of thought. For instance, when I started to introduce you to our group, I couldn't, for the life of me, remember the name of the girl who had just joined our team two days ago. When I finally sat down in the bathroom just now, I went 'Tally! Her name's Tally.' What was wrong with me? It frightens me. I used to be very sharp and on it." Courtney frowned and shook her head.

"I think it's not only the chemo with me, but I think it's also all the surgeries I've had. My sister [a younger sister who is a pediatrician] said that some of the stuff used for general anesthesia can cause what amounts to amnesia. I'm not sure—I may be saying it wrong, because I'm not a medical person—but I think all of the surgeries, going under general anesthesia all those times, and the chemo have caused my brain to be mushy at times ... I'll reach for milk in the refrigerator and I'll drop it. It's like my brain can't tell my hand to hang on tight enough. The right messages aren't going through. I had CMF [combination chemotherapy], and one of them, I think, fried my brain. All the girls in my young survivors' groups joked about chemo brain. We've been calling it chemo brain since 1996. Now, I read studies about it, and I'm like, yeah, we knew."

One of the first studies that linked cognitive dysfunction and chemotherapy treatment for breast cancer was reported in 1995; subsequent studies have supported those findings. For some women, the cognitive impairment experienced during chemotherapy treatment is reversible, while others continue to have problems with memory, concentration, and so-called "executive skills"—the ability to process multiple disparate thoughts and synthesize cogent ideas. As Courtney intimated, neurotoxicity ("chemo brain") can be a significant problem for some patients that persists for years after completing treatment.

She continued. "In a way, it's made me understand what my special ed students go through when they are trying to retrieve something from a mental file and can't find it back in there. I know exactly what that's like now—that retrieval process. That was something, as a straight-A student, that I never had to deal with before. I now completely understand what they're going through, and understand their learning difficulties a little bit better now."

Being a special education teacher was Courtney's second career. Her first was screen acting. She said, "All I wanted to do when I was growing up in Atwater, California, was come to LA and be like Hayley Mills and be in Disney movies." After finishing high school, she attended the University of California at Irvine and graduated in three years with a Bachelor of Arts degree in theater, winning the Miss Atwater crown along the way. Then it was on to Hollywood. She acted in four horror films: *Killing Spree, Slaughterhouse, Things,* and *Feast.* "I did low-budget films. I had a blast. I had so much fun. There's nothing like finally getting a part in a movie, no matter how silly it is. Especially with horror films, people have a really good sense of humor because they're just so silly. I loved doing horror films. It was fun, but they all wanted you to take your clothes off, and I just wouldn't do it. I wouldn't have done it differently. It's just who I am. I don't put down people who can take their clothes off, but it's just not me, and I couldn't imagine my family seeing me naked, like in a love scene with somebody, or doing one of those silly teen-age movies taking my clothes off. I just couldn't do it.

"I did all of these horror films and refused to take my clothes off—which is a joke with God because now, all I ever do is go in and take my clothes off for people." Courtney rolled her eyes and laughed. "For my mastectomy, they took nude pictures of me—nude pictures of my butt, of my boobs. I would never do that for acting ... I have a scar from here down to here all the way across both sides, under both arms. My stomach, my belly button, down here. I'm scarred everywhere. I'm Sally, The Patchwork Girl, from Tim Burton's *Nightmare Before Christmas*." Courtney tried to point out the scars, but the pink, fluffy wings that she was wearing got in her way.

The scars that she was describing resulted from surgical treatment and reconstruction for bilateral breast cancer—the first diagnosis in October 1996; the second in June 1998. She discovered the first while showering in May 1996 and saw her primary care physician the following month. He ordered a mammogram, which was negative and, subsequently, an ultrasound, which was also negative. Still, he referred her to a surgeon who, at Courtney's request, did a biopsy the same day as the intake visit. "I told the surgeon that I had just started a new job. I was in a special teaching program, and I needed to quit having all these appointments. I didn't have the money to pay for the parking, the co-payments. I said, 'Let's just get it over with.' So he did the excision that day under local anesthesia. When he showed me the tumor, he said that it was fine—it didn't have irregular edges, or whatever. He said, 'I'm sure that it's probably nothing.'

"Then, I got the call a few days later saying that it was something ... I was in my classroom at the school where I teach [Marquez Charter Elementary School in Pacific Palisades]. Since I was a special education teacher, I had a phone in my room. I got my diagnosis, and I remember walking out the door and just crying hysterically going into the office. I hadn't even told my family about this because I thought it was nothing ... The nurse didn't exactly tell me over the phone, she just said, 'You can't come by yourself. You have to bring somebody.' I said, 'I went in for the local surgery by myself. Why am I bringing somebody in for the follow-up?' And she repeated, 'You must not come in alone for the results of the biopsy.'

"That was it. She didn't have to say it. I knew right then that I had cancer ... We talk about that a lot in support groups and also in discussions with the Young Survival Coalition® [members] that I meet. How were you told? What did they do? Did they call you? Did they tell you when you came in? Were you alone? There's really no ideal way to tell somebody."

As Courtney had feared, the surgeon told her that her biopsy results were positive for infiltrating ductal carcinoma and that the tumor extended to the margin of the biopsy. She said, "The whole thing is a blur for the first time because I was so upset and angry. They had told me so many times that I didn't have it, that when they finally told me that I did have it, I was in complete denial. I said, 'I don't have it. I'm going to call the producers of *Oprah* and *60 Minutes*. I want them to follow my biopsy tissue to pathology. I think they switched my slides. I've got the wrong diagnosis.'

"I was pretty numb through that whole part. A lot of information went in one ear and out the other, because I was convinced that I didn't have cancer. They *told* me I didn't. I had a mammogram, and I didn't have it. I had an ultrasound, and I didn't have it. There was no way. I was 33 years old. No one in my family had breast cancer. I wasn't a smoker. I'm not a drinker. I eat healthy. I'm from a very healthy family. Everyone lives very long lives. There was no way that I had breast cancer.

"In my support group, they teased me about it. They would say, 'You were the girl that was going through chemo but didn't have cancer.' It took me a long time to accept it. When the psychosocial [team member] wrote her report for the UCLA [University of California at Los Angeles] multidisciplinary clinic, it was along the lines of 'Watch out for her psychosocially,' because I was such a mess. I seriously wanted to call Dan Rather, or whomever, and say, 'Please follow somebody from the time they have their biopsy until they put it on the slides, because they mixed mine up.' I was very adamant about it."

The UCLA clinic that she mentioned was the Revlon/UCLA Breast Center at UCLA's Jonsson Cancer Center, where she was referred for treatment. Although multidisciplinary centers like the Revlon/UCLA Breast Center are now fairly common; in 1996, when she was diagnosed, clinics of this type were in their infancy. To facilitate her evaluation, Courtney's mother, who had also gone with her to the follow-up appointment, drove around Los Angles to collect the imaging studies and pathology slides—the ones that Courtney was convinced were someone else's. The diagnostic part of the team (a pathologist and a radiologist) reviewed this material before Courtney and her mother met with the treatment part of the team (a surgeon, a medical oncologist, a radiation oncologist, and a psychologist).

She ultimately underwent a wide local excision and axillary dissection, followed by four cycles of Adriamycin® and Cytoxan® and radiation treatment. "I still had trouble believing that I had breast cancer ... Losing my hair was hard. My hair was this long, maybe even longer." She pointed to her long brown hair that hung halfway down her back. "The first time around with A/C—just like they promised me—on December 15, it was just out of there. That was devastating ... I was completely bald. I always wore a cap. I only took the cap off to take a shower. I got into the shower. I took off my hat after I got in. I put the hat right back on. I slept in the hat." She covered her eyes with both hands, bowed her head, and added, "I just couldn't have it in my face that I was going through this.

"I wouldn't talk to anybody about it. I didn't accept any help. Teachers offered to give me their sick days so that I wouldn't have to use all my sick days, offered to cook meals for me, offered to help me with my daughter. I was a single mom with a three-year-old daughter at the time. I wouldn't accept any help except from one family that picked up Sedona [her daughter] every Thursday from preschool and kept her for the rest of the afternoon and the evening while I went to school for special ed credentials and for my support group after that. They did that for me for almost a year. That was the only real help, besides my family, my immediate family, that I would accept. I wouldn't accept phone calls. I wouldn't talk to people." Courtney pressed her lips together. She walked in silence for a minute or so, perhaps reflecting on how angry and isolated she had felt.

"I was angry. I was devastated. I would think, Why me? Some of my friends work for companies and make all this money. I'm a teacher. I don't make all that much money. I'm a good person. I'm in special ed. I like to help children. There are people who say, 'Why *not* me?' but I've always wanted to know, 'Why me? Why would this happen to me?' The second time I was diagnosed with infiltrating ductal carcinoma—on the other side, another primary tumor—was when it finally sunk in that I had it.

"Even though it was only a year and a half later, I was able to do the sentinel node biopsy, which made things a lot better. They didn't get clear margins for the first lumpectomy, tried again, still couldn't get clear margins. That second attempt at getting clear margins, they found more cancer—DCIS [ductal carcinoma *in situ*], and I think they found another tumor—so the surgeon said, 'We have to do a mastectomy.' That threw me for a loop *again*. I was finally okay with the fact that, alright, I guess I really did have cancer the first time. I've got it again, the second time, and I'm going in for a lumpectomy. I'm going to have chemo and radiation, and I'm going to be done. Lose my hair again, whatever, but then, after two lumpectomies, they tell me I'm going to have to have a *mastectomy*. That really threw me for a loop."

Before Courtney had her mastectomy, though, she plugged into her favorite coping outlet and left for an overseas vacation. Less than five years before, when she and her first husband split up, she had traveled to Thailand alone. She was three months pregnant. This time, dreading a mastectomy, she and her mother went to Budapest. About leaving her first husband, she said, "I packed up and got out of there, with nothing, no money, no nothing. I had a little beta fish—this Chinese fighting fish—in my car on the console and drove home from Vegas with my car packed. I had a couple of weeks before I was going to start a long-term teaching position … I didn't know where I was going to live when I got back, but I just took off and went to Thailand for two weeks."

For the trip to Budapest, she packed one of Dr. Bernie Segal's books about self-healing. "It talked a lot about using your mind to try and heal yourself ... It was just really a positive book for me, an uplifting book for me. I would try and try and try to do the centipede game with my tumor to try to get rid of it. I would tell my mom, 'I'm trying and trying, but I can't get rid of it. It just won't go away.' So I came back, and I knew that I had to get the mastectomy.

"I did a lot of searches. Was I going to do an implant? Was I going to do a flap? What was I going to do? I finally went with the flap, because so many women that I talked to with an implant had to go back for more surgery within five years because it burst or leaked or whatever. By this point, I'd had so many surgeries, and my veins were so bad from all the chemo, that I felt like I couldn't keep having additional surgeries ... I was thinner at the time, and I couldn't do a TRAM flap [transverse rectus abdominis myocutaneous flap reconstruction], so my choices were the thigh or the back or the butt. I didn't want my back with a huge scar all the way down. I liked my back. So I decided I'd do the butt.

"It almost killed me going through the gluteal flap reconstruction. It wasn't a problem with the doctor; it was that my jugular vein wasn't taking the blood out as quickly as the arteries were bringing it in, and I kept getting a hematoma. I had complications from the beginning—my sister would know about it. I was in surgery from 7 in the morning until 10 o'clock at night—a very, very, very long time. Then I came out, and they'd put me in recovery, and the only thing I remember—it was at UCLA at the teaching hospital—was all the little interns coming in. I remember a girl and a guy, and they're looking over me, and I'm barely coming to, and they're saying, 'Omigod, what do we do?' They're completely freaking out. They're trying to keep cool, but my breast is completely blown up with this hematoma, and they're saying, 'We have to call! We have to call the doctor!'" Courtney pumped her fists in front of her chest, imitating the panic of the doctors-in-training.

"So they brought the surgeon back in, without calling my family, for another emergency surgery to deal with the hematoma. All my family is at my house, 7 o'clock in the morning, getting ready to come to the hospital, thinking they're coming to see me in recovery, and they get a phone call. 'We're bringing her in again for the third time. She had a big hematoma. It happened again.'

"They said, 'The *third* time?'

"And the nurse said, 'Yeah, we had to take her back again in the middle of the night. She's going in again.'

"So my family comes to the hospital, and they're completely beside themselves, because I've just come out of the *third* surgery. My mom; my dad; my stepdad; both my sisters; my brother; my girlfriend, Terry; my boyfriend, Ron, who is now my husband, and whom I'd just met two weeks before my mastectomy. Ron was there through this whole thing. That's how he got to know my family—when I was in the hospital this whole time.

"Finally, they cut these slits all the way down my neck, and they took my jugular vein and tunneled it down, and I have a piece of my rib taken out here." She pointed to her lower rib cage. "They moved my jugular vein to ..." She looked down at her chest, squinted, said, "Hmmm ...," then added, "I don't know where it is. I've been through the ringer. You thought I was angry the first time? I think I was in surgery for something like 21 hours in a 48-hour period. It was *huge* what I was going through. It was a nightmare."

As if a second breast cancer, a mastectomy, and life-threatening surgical complications weren't enough body punches, a disturbing situation involving her ex-husband surfaced shortly before she was to begin chemotherapy for the second time. She was almost overwhelmed with anger and frustration during this period of her life; however, when we walked together, it was clear that she had somehow mastered these emotions, averted bitterness and hatred, and had, in fact, achieved peacefulness.

She said the turning point occurred when she was lying in bed and saw Jesus and angels on the ceiling of the room. The image was so vivid that it allowed her to relinquish much of her anger. "It was very specific the way that Jesus looked. Most of the time in representations of Christ in churches, his arms are out or his arms are up. The Jesus that came to me had his arms down and his hands were out like this, in a white robe. I was just in Paris this summer with a girlfriend at the [Basilique du] Sacre-Coeur and the [statue of] Jesus there was the exact Jesus that came to me. It was very bizarre to see it again, and I just stood there and started crying. My girlfriend, Nynette, wrote down what it said next to the statue. That's why angels are a very big deal in my life."

She was referring to her 3-Day team's name—Team Pink Wings—as well as her Web site—Pink Wings 4 Breast Cancer (www.pinkwings.com)—through which she markets breast cancer awareness items that are geared towards younger buyers. "I try to make cool, beautiful items so that the 20-year-olds are wearing them, teen-agers are wearing them, everyone's wearing them, with the hope that people will realize that young people get this disease, too. You can't always wear a shirt that screams breast cancer awareness with a big pink ribbon on it. You can't slam everyone in the face with shirts.

"We do cute little shirts with tiny little crystals—very subtle. The jewelry we do is also very subtle. The pins we do are more fun and more subtle. We just try to be different. We design all of the clothing and the pins. I don't design the jewelry, but I select items that I like that aren't on the other Web sites. We try it out and wear it to make sure we like the way it wears. I want everybody wearing a pink ribbon, because everyone's affected by it."

Her advocacy has gone well beyond long-distance walks and her Web site business. She served on the Steering Committee and chaired the Survivor Committee for the inaugural Pacific Palisades American Cancer Society Relay For Life®. She has participated in the Revlon Run/Walk for Women® and Expedition Inspiration's Help Breast Cancer Take-a-Hike® events, and she was one of 20 breast cancer survivors nationwide who were selected to participate in an Adventure Weekend, sponsored by Girl Teams in Los Angeles. She has also volunteered with the American Cancer Society's Reach to Recovery® program.

"When I'm talking to a newly diagnosed person, I have to put myself back into the frame of mind that I had. When I was diagnosed, Reach to Recovery® called me, and I wouldn't even return phone calls. I never spoke to a person, so I have to remember what it was like then. They certainly don't need to hear about going through it twice, but it's hard to avoid mentioning that, because going through it twice is so much of who I am."

Courtney also spoke of national media opportunities that resulted from being a breast cancer survivor. The first was a photograph of her wearing a cap (to cover her near-bald head), holding her daughter, Sedona, which appeared in the 1998 brochure for the Revlon Run/Walk for Women®, right below a picture of Oprah Winfrey. The photograph had been taken at the 1997 event, shortly after Courtney finished chemotherapy for her first breast cancer. She was also in a nationally televised Ford commercial about finding a cure for breast cancer, and was one of the featured survivors on an original seven-part series for the International Channel entitled, "Sharing Hope, Facing Breast Cancer." And last, but certainly not least in her mind, was the chance to meet Donny Osmond.

"All my life, I was in love with Donny Osmond. I remember being a little girl in Atwater, California, and I remember standing up in a little outfit and making my mom take a picture of me to send to a teen magazine to win a chance to meet Donny Osmond. So I get breast cancer, and I start doing a lot of speaking for the Avon 3-Days—I was on the media team. They put us on the *Leeza Gibbons Show*, and I said to the girl, 'If you ever get a chance to do the *Donny & Marie Show*'—they had a talk show at the time, too—'please keep me in mind.' Omigod, I've always wanted to meet Donny. Within a few days, she called me up and said, 'Are you sitting down? We're going on the *Donny & Marie Show* next week, and you're on.' I got to sit in the green room and talk with him. I got an Avon Breast Cancer 3-Day shirt that's autographed by him that's in my closet in a little canvas bag with my precious dresses. And I have a picture that was taken with him."

Courtney shrugged her shoulders and laughed. "I guess it just happens at the time it's supposed to happen. I'm filmed constantly; I'm interviewed for newspapers constantly; I was in a full-page ad in *Self* magazine last October for the Avon Walk for Breast Cancer—wearing a shirt that said, 'Great Breasts (They were diagnosed early!)' ... I tried to do acting for so long, and I just couldn't do it. Finally, when I was pregnant, I decided I needed to give up that dream for a while, because I needed to raise money for my kid, so I got into teaching. It took getting breast cancer. I mean, that's the whole reason that all of this stuff started coming to me.

"Did you read the Lance Armstrong book? At the very beginning of the book, when he was diagnosed, he got an e-mail from a guy whom he didn't know. The guy said to him, 'You don't know it yet, but you've just been given a gift.' I read the book this summer, and I totally knew what that guy was talking about. So I take it as a gift now, and I feel like if I had it to do again, I don't think I would have it be different. I don't think I would have ever come on one of these walks if I hadn't been diagnosed." She motioned toward the walkers ahead of us and added, "I don't know if this would have been a part of my life. I've met wonderful people, and I can't imagine my life not having those people in it. Lots of my best friends are from my survivor group.

"Another thing that happened was that Ron's [her second husband's] mom was diagnosed with breast cancer the second time when I was diagnosed; we lost her just a few years ago, in August. We used to walk in support of her; now we walk in her memory. She and I were going through chemo together. We lived just a few doors down from each other, so it was really nice. I think she felt really good being able to talk about things, and I felt really good being able to talk to her about it ... She loved me, and I loved her. She was just a wonderful, sweet person."

Still, Courtney did not trivialize the costs of having breast cancer at a young age. "The worst part about having cancer is having your fertility taken away. It's been so wonderful to meet all the young survivors, to meet up with the Young Survival Coalition® out of New York, which is the most wonderful organization in the world for us young survivors. They understand how it makes me feel when people who haven't had cancer look at me and say, 'Well, but you're still alive. You can't have more children, but you have your daughter.' Even if I didn't have a child, those same people would say, 'Whatever. You're alive, and that's all that matters.' That's *not* all that matters, because when I came on this earth, I thought I was going to get married and have a whole bunch of kids, but that was taken away from me. I want to tell those people, 'Yes, I am alive, but I still want more children.'"

A couple of years after she and Ron were married (on July 4, 2000), they decided to pursue adoption. Ron's hope was to adopt a child, but Courtney had other plans. "I had identical twin cousins, so ever since I was a little girl, I wanted to be a twin. I'd watch *Parent Trap*, and I would go to bed and cry, because I wanted to be a twin so badly. I wanted to grow up and have twins ... We hired an attorney to try to adopt, and we asked him about getting twins. Part of the reason was that Ron is older. He just turned 51, and he had never been married, and never had kids before." Courtney laughed and added, "Another reason was that I knew I wanted more than one more kid, and if I was going to get two, I'd better get two at once, because he might not let me get a second one after we had one."

She and Ron didn't adopt biological twins; however, they adopted infant girls who were born within weeks of one another. Their names are Sage and Sienna, and Courtney and Ron call them "the twins." Ron brought the twins and their older sister, Sedona, to camp on Day 2 to visit their mommy. Sedona's hair was short, because she had recently donated 16 inches of her hair to Locks of Love at the Pacific Palisades Relay For Life®, raising $2,000 in pledges for the American Cancer Society. Locks of Love is a nonprofit organization that provides hairpieces for financially disadvantaged children. The two-year-olds were in their double stroller and they looked, if not like identical twins, certainly enough alike to be fraternal twins. They looked like two little angels.

Although Courtney had longed for more children, her concern about recurrence intensified during the time that she and Ron were considering adoption. "I thought, If it's in my brain, it's bad, and I won't be around to take care of these kids. I didn't tell anybody, but I went in for a brain MRI. While I waited for those results—omigod—it was awful. It was *excruciating* waiting for the results. I'd had my CBC [complete blood count] done and my mammogram and my CA 27-29." (CA 27-29 is a cancer antigen that is similar to CA 15-3.)

Fortunately, all of her studies were normal—she didn't have metastatic disease in her brain, after all—so she and Ron proceeded with adopting their twin daughters. As mentioned at the beginning of this section, though, Courtney still thinks about recurrence nearly every day.

In contrast to Courtney, Carol Schwartz, 46, said that she was rarely concerned about recurrence. "I'm the type of person who doesn't like to anticipate problems and spend time worrying about something that might happen or could be. I have enough things to do to deal with as it is. I hate it when my husband does it. I tell him, 'Is there anything we can do about it?' That's not to say that I have the attitude of, 'So what.' I'm taking much better care of myself. I'll eat better food, and that sort of thing, but I'm not going to allow myself to get paralyzed by concern about recurrence."

Actually, her pragmatism is not misguided. The results of two multicenter studies involving almost 2,500 women showed that there was no difference in overall survival between women who received intensive surveillance and those who had physical exams and only clinically indicated tests. Put another way, if an asymptomatic breast cancer survivor underwent frequent bone scans, liver echography, chest x-rays, and laboratory tests, her recurrence was *detected* a month or two earlier than it otherwise would have been, but it didn't influence how long she survived. Put still another way: Why waste time and money when all you achieve is a false sense of security?

Carol had reached the same conclusions without the benefit of robust studies. To make the point, she described a typical conversation with Dr. Linnea Chap, her medical oncologist, during a follow-up appointment since completing chemotherapy. (Carol's rendition of the conversation was hilarious because she paused dramatically between each line and exaggerated her native New York accent.)

"Hello, Dr. Chap."

"Hello, Carol. How are you?"

"I'm fine."

"How are you feeling?"

"Fine."

"Okay, you can get dressed now."

Carol laughed and continued. "Then we chat about her kids or my kids, because there's nothing they can do about a recurrence. There are no blood tests that they can perform that are a precise way to screen for recurrence. If they don't feel a lump, if they don't catch something on a mammogram, there's nothing that they can do, so I think it's almost comical that I have to go in and do all of that."

Carol's first opportunity to be levelheaded about breast cancer arose when she had a routine mammogram in July 2003. The studies were suspicious for ductal carcinoma in situ [DCIS], which prompted stereotactic biopsies that supported this diagnosis. Her gynecologist referred her to a surgeon at Cedars-Sinai Medical Center in Los Angeles. "I had two lumpectomies done at the same time to try to remove where the DCIS seemed to be most concentrated. Neither of the lumpectomies had clear margins and, in one of them, they found a 0.6 cm invasive tumor. They said, 'We can try and do more lumpectomies, which will probably disfigure you, but we recommend instead that you have a mastectomy.'"

One of Carol's friends, whose mother had died of breast cancer, was being closely monitored through the High Risk Program at the Revlon/UCLA Breast Center. She suggested that Carol consider evaluation through the Breast Cancer Multidisciplinary Program. "She recommended the nurse practitioner who runs the program there. She said that I had to get a second opinion, and she got me into the second-opinion program real quickly and also got me an appointment with the head surgeon at UCLA. At the second opinion, they said, 'Yeah, you need a mastectomy. The diagnosis was correct.' Then I met with Dr. Helena Chang, and she said, 'You've got to do this.' (Dr. Chang is the director of the Revlon/UCLA Breast Center.)

"I really, really liked the treatment that I was getting there—the fact that it was comprehensive. While I was going through my private doctors, who all had operating privileges at Cedars-Sinai—I mean, not shabby care—I had to physically carry my stuff. I just didn't feel like it was coordinated very well, especially when they started talking about referrals to plastic surgeons and chemotherapy and all this other stuff. I said, 'No, I'm going for one-stop shopping.'"

She ultimately had a mastectomy and low axillary node dissection (15 nodes) with an immediate TRAM flap reconstruction. "They found no more invasive cancer. I had DCIS. That one lump that was removed during the lumpectomy—the 0.6 cm one—was the only one that was invasive. The pathology of the tumor was estrogen-receptor negative and *HER-2/neu* positive, which meant that I would not be a candidate for tamoxifen. Given my age, there was a question about whether or not to do chemo. I was referred to Dr. Chap, who was also at UCLA, for my medical oncology treatment. In the end, she erred on the conservative side—to treat me more aggressively, as opposed to less aggressively. We agreed on a treatment of Adriamycin® and Cytoxan®. We agreed to do four minimum, and then to see how I was handling it. If my body was not totally abused by it, to then do a couple more. I ended up with six, and my last treatment was January 30 [2004].

"As part of the comprehensive health care that you get at UCLA, I met with a social worker a couple of times. She told me, 'I know from your time commitments, you're not going to participate in a support group, but if you should decide to do that, it's available.' I tend to compartmentalize things. What I'm doing with my health wasn't really affecting other things in my life so much. I would just put it in its own box in my head. Emotionally, that's how I did it.

"I shared a lot with my friends and my family, and I had a lot of support from people who I never thought would rise to the occasion, but they did. For instance, people who were just acquaintances would leave dinner in a bag outside our door. Or my brother, who works in New York and lives in New Jersey, flew out to make sure he was there when I was having surgery. So people did a lot of things."

Her ability to, as she described, "compartmentalize things"—which I took to mean approaching a problem in a logical, stepwise fashion, considering only *relevant* information—may have ties to her educational background. After finishing public high school in New York City (skipping eighth grade along the way), she entered MIT [Massachusetts Institute of Technology] as a mathematics major, but soon switched to architecture. "I have my Bachelor of Science in architecture, and stayed there and got my master's in architecture. I practiced architecture for about five or six years and then decided to go back to school to get my MBA [Master in Business Administration degree]. I went to Harvard for my MBA and graduated in '89. Now I do consulting in real estate development."

It was while she was attending MIT that she met her future husband, Steven Drucker. "He went to Harvard for architecture, but we met at MIT because he was cross-registering. We married a year after I got my master's in architecture ... My husband and I had both worked in Boston for a long time. We didn't like anything about the winter in Boston except to leave there and go on vacation to the Caribbean, so we decided it would probably be a good idea to relocate. We came to Los Angeles. I had a job, and then he got a job, and we've been here ever since ... Now that we have kids, it's kind of sad that they're not near their cousins, but we have a great life out here. We love where we are. The kids have a good school. We wouldn't go back."

Carol and Steven's daughter, Micki, was five years old, and their son, Charlie, was eight years old when she was diagnosed. Again, Carol showed her true stripes when she considered how she and Steven would approach telling their children about her cancer. "I talked to the pediatrician. I did some research over at UCLA. Everybody basically says to tell them whatever they're capable of understanding, don't get into too much detail, and sort of gauge what they can accept. So we told them. We also wanted to say 'cancer,' because we didn't want them to hear it from someone else.

"We told them that I had breast cancer and that I had some really good doctors and that I was going to be okay, but that I was going to have to have some surgery and maybe some chemotherapy and that I was going to lose my hair, but it wasn't going to be a problem. My son and daughter are very different. My son was like, 'Yeah, yeah, yeah, okay.' My daughter wanted to talk about it a lot. We told their teachers what was going on so they'd know to watch for changes in their behavior.

"When I'd go to my daughter's classroom, she'd take me over to her teacher and say, 'My mommy's right breast is sick.' Then, when I was going through chemo, she'd say, 'Mommy's wearing a wig. Do you want to see her head?' She was just very, very verbal." Carol laughed and shook her head. "That was fine, because I didn't have anything that I was hiding.

"Charlie, on the other hand, didn't really talk about it. After I got home from the hospital, some balloons were delivered to the house. One of the balloons said, 'Sorry you're under the weather.' My son asked, 'Why does the balloon say that?' I said, 'Maybe you don't understand the saying.' He said, 'No, I know what it means. It means that you don't feel well. Just because you have breast cancer means you don't feel well?'

"So I thought, fine. Cool. I think they've handled it very well." Carol laughed again.

Carol said that her husband may have been the family member who was most concerned about the situation. "He was probably more worried about me when I was going through surgery than I was. At this point, he doesn't talk to me about that he's worried about me. It could be one of two reasons. He knows that I just don't want to hear it. Again, what are you going to do about it? Or, it could be that I've not let it impact me in a way where I'm less of who I was than before, and it isn't so much on his mind."

Or, maybe, I suggested, that her ability to train for a 60-mile walk helped ease his mind. Maybe her participation was one of his ways of coping with the anxiety that his wife might develop a recurrence. She smiled slowly at the suggestion, and answered, nodding, "Maybe. Maybe so."

It was actually Carol's husband who had urged her to participate in the 3-Day. "When I was in the hospital, my husband found a brochure for the 3-Day at UCLA. He showed it to me, and he said, 'I think you can do this.' I said no, because I'd never been very athletic, but he said, 'No, no, no. I think you can.' He mentioned it a few times, and I told him that I'd look into it. He felt, for me, it would be a good way to get through it and heal. He really encouraged me."

Carol raised over $10,000 and was one of the top fundraisers for the Los Angeles 3-Day. "My husband said that yesterday morning my daughter said to him, 'I'm really glad mommy's doing this walk. It's really good for her, and it's really good for a lot of other people, too.'"

One of those "other people" who benefits from the 3-Day walk and the other fundraising endeavors of the Susan G. Komen Foundation is, of course, Carol's daughter. And my daughter. All our daughters. And our sons. All of us. Every single one of us. *Every single one of us on this planet.*

I don't want to stand accused of kissing anyone's boots (to mix and mangle metaphors), so I'll skip the recitation of staggering numbers—besides, if you're interested, the how-many-millions information is on their Web site (www.komen.org)—but the Susan G. Komen Foundation has (and is) doing good work. Period.

Detractors accuse the Komen Foundation of not allocating enough money for this or not directing enough money toward that. For instance, an article forwarded to me accused the Komen Foundation of not channeling enough research money to investigate the epidemiology of breast cancer. Sure, we all want that puzzle solved, but charging the Komen Foundation with dereliction of their research duties aggravated me.

The Komen Foundation Award and Research Grant Program observes a stringent review process, so that the contributions—including the $3.2 million raised by the 1,140 Los Angeles 3-Day walkers—isn't wasted on poorly designed, redundant, underpowered, or just plain stupid studies. So, to the detractors, I say this: "*Shut up!* You obviously aren't medically sophisticated enough to know what you're griping about." (Up until this point, I have tried to be winsome and demure, but I'm getting near the end of the book and frankly, I needed to get that off what's left of my chest.)

Besides funding research, Komen also sponsors educational and awareness initiatives. One of these is an online, interactive tutorial about breast cancer and an animated instructional guide for breast self-exams. This material is the centerpiece for *On the Way to the Cure—Komen on the Go®*, a traveling tour that visits college and university campuses as well as community events. The colorful cruiser, outfitted with laptops, visited some of the 2004 3-Day events, including Los Angeles, where I had a chance to watch the instructional guide and take the tutorial. I missed one of the questions on the self-test but, after reviewing the material, eventually got it right.

Nearly everyone who walked for Barbara Jo and Bob Kirshbaum's Team California visited the tour cruiser and went online for the tutorial and guide, including Debra Johnson, Ronda Starkenburg, and David Kirshbaum, who are Barbara Jo and Bob's grown children; and their friends Randi, Michelle, Sarah, and Andrea. The tutorial, which stressed early detection, was instructive for all age groups, but it was aimed at younger women, like the majority of Team California.

David Kirshbaum is a physician's assistant with his father's internal medicine practice, so he watched it as an educational exercise and also to be a good sport. Outnumbered by the women on his team, David functioned as the one-man equivalent of Boston's Men With Heart, beginning at Opening Ceremonies at Huntington State Beach, all the way through to Closing Ceremonies at Santa Monica Pier.

If I were to summarize the Los Angeles 3-Day route, it would be wide zigzags to and from the beach: away from the beach, back to the beach, along the beach, away from the beach, back to the beach, along the beach, etc. Day 1's zigzag was mainly in Huntington Beach; Day 2's was in Long Beach; Day 3's was in Santa Monica (after a relatively straight-shot early morning bus ride to Day 3's departure point at Marina del Rey). By the end of Day 2, after walking nearly 43 miles (and even retracing some of our steps on Day 1), we were only 15 miles closer to our endpoint than when we had started. But we had made progress. We were closer.

That characterization of our journey is not a criticism. In fact, it serves as a metaphor for this chapter's theme: concern about recurrence. We who have had breast cancer zigzag to and from our pacific beach, hopefully making a little progress, but sometimes we have to retrace our steps. I'll wager that even women and men as wise as Carol Schwartz have occasional tremors.

Since I was an honorary member of Team California and, for that matter, the Kirshbaum family (as Barbara Jo's "adopted" sister), I walked much of the Los Angeles 3-Day event with this remarkable group, laughing most of the time; however, when Ronda Starkenburg and I walked together, she shared why she became involved with the 3-Day and began raising money for the breast cancer cause. Unlike her mother, Barbara Jo, who initially participated in long-distance walks for the physical challenge, Ronda had a personal reason for becoming involved. A close friend, Theresa Vela, died from breast cancer at age 36, just six weeks after walking in the 2002 Los Angeles 3-Day. Ronda now designs, assembles, and sells pink-ribbon-themed jewelry, donating a large percentage of her profits.

Along the route on Day 3, I met Ronda's husband, Chris, and their daughters, Allie and Maddie. Like Sedona Zinszer, Allie Starkenburg, 6, had recently donated her hair to Locks of Love, and her younger sister, Maddie, 4, was planning to donate her hair as soon as it was long enough. The two little girls walked part of the route on Day 3 with their mother, aunt, uncle, and grandmother. Fittingly, it was Maddie Starkenburg who closed the angel arc that had begun at the Los Angeles Opening Ceremonies. Let me retrace that arc.

When we arrived for Opening Ceremonies, the weather looked like the set for one of Courtney's horror movies: dark, misty, and chilly. Locals called the thick fog the "marine layer" and assured nonlocals that it would lift mid-morning—which it did, at exactly 10:25 AM on Day 1. But at 6 AM, despite the customary loud, upbeat music and the bright lights, the crowd's mood was somewhat subdued.

Enter stage left: two large-boned women dressed as angels, complete with halos, wings, and long, shimmering robes that billowed as they walked. They were sweep crew members, but the sight of these women, with their semitranslucent robes back-lit by the stage lights, was ethereal. As they floated toward us, we nudged one another and giggled: The angels were smoking cigarettes. The fog remained, but the mood miraculously lifted.

The midpoint of the arc was during the walk, of course, when Courtney told me about her vision of angels and Jesus—a vision that brought her peace and comfort. In other words, she talked about actual angels.

Finally, as I waited for Closing Ceremonies and took my nap, another type of angel appeared. The grass in the holding area was thick and mushy, and there was a soothing breeze off the bay. Out of earshot of the loud music, I slept more soundly than usual, only to awake to a cherubic face, leaning over me and smiling. She whispered, "They said I should tell you to wake up." She handed me a rose and ran away.

I sat up and yelled after her, "Thank you, Maddie!" She kept running toward her family, all of them looking in my direction, laughing and waving. I waved back. *Los angeles*, indeed.

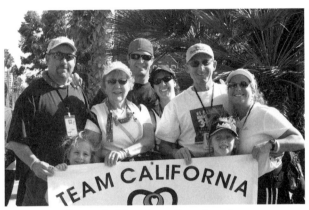

Team California at Los Angeles

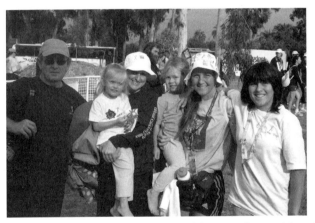

Courtney Lercara-Zinszer, second from right, and her family

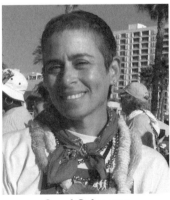

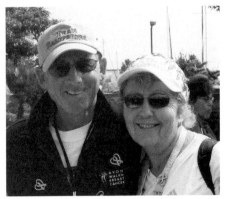

Carol Schwartz   *Bob and Barbara Jo Kirshbaum*

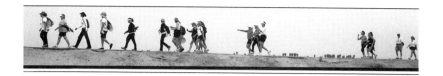

Chapter 9

San Francisco
October 15, October 16, and October 17, 2004

Peripheral vision sharpens when you unfold your trail map and discover that you're halfway up Bear Mountain; or you're sitting cross-legged on a big, flat rock in Rattlesnake Canyon; or the secluded path you're on is alongside Panther Creek. Even back in the days of tie-dyed shirts and incense—when I did authentic camping—it was still a bummer to discover that I'd crashed on Porcupine Bluff.

Knowing the names of the places where I am hiking (or, for that matter, walking in an urban jungle) is less about potential creature encounters than connecting the dots: I was there, now I'm here; if I go this way, I won't get lost because I'm going to be there, right *there*. Even if the chance of getting lost is minimal—like, for instance, when I was among 1,607 walkers at the San Francisco 3-Day—I still prefer to know the names of my destinations, even if those names don't mean diddly to me. Unfortunately, the San Francisco route cards didn't include the exact locations of the Pit Stops and Grab & Go stations. I spent much of the event, more or less, lost—at least in terms of knowing the name of the dot.

As was the case at other events, San Francisco's Day 1 route card was distributed after Opening Ceremonies, and Day 2 and 3 cards were distributed as we left camp each morning. The cards were 2 by 4 inches and, as mentioned in Chapter 1, fit snuggly in the credentials sleeve that we wore around our necks. The little cards listed the mileage and the closing times of each of the rest stops, and, for *every* event except San Francisco and Arizona, they also listed the *exact names* of the rest stops—often a city park, a school yard, a church parking lot, or some other flat, open area adjacent to a public institution that could accommodate supply stations, porta-potties, and a waiting sweep bus or van.

At first, it troubled me that I didn't know where I was going until I got there in San Francisco—that I didn't know the *label* of the next dot—but, by the afternoon of Day 1, I decided to trust the other walkers to usher me along and to live in the moment, not worrying about the particulars of our destination.

It was apt that I was walking with Karen Schweibish, 50, a breast cancer survivor from Manhattan Beach (near Los Angeles), because she was nearly as clueless as I was about our whereabouts in the San Francisco Bay Area. She, too, talked about the importance (and challenge) of living in the moment. Interestingly, it wasn't the diagnosis of breast cancer but an ankle fracture that she sustained while undergoing chemotherapy that first caused her to reflect on this.

She described the incident. "I was taking the garbage out, and I didn't have a wig on, which was fine. I had just had a chemo treatment and I just looked nasty. I was pale, and I was not in a good state. You know that show, *Survivor?*" I shrugged and shook my head. She continued. "Where the people go to an island and have to survive for a month?" I shook my head again.

She smiled and said, "You really don't watch TV, do you? Whatever. Well, my whole family loved that show, and it was the final episode, so they were all watching it, but the garbage was bothering me, so I wanted to take it out. I had on a pair of platform shoes." She must have seen my surprise because she added, "I know, I know. It was dumb. Anyway, I saw a neighbor walking his dog, and I thought, Omigod, he's going to want to talk to me, and I don't want to talk to him. I didn't look good, and I didn't feel good, so I started to run with my garbage, and I did one of these off-the-side-of-my-shoe-onto-my-ankle things." Karen shuddered and shook her head.

"I really felt like I needed to slow down, and it was God's way of saying—I'm not even a religious person—but it was God's message that I don't live in the present. I am running like a crazy person, and I really needed to slow down, and He was going to make sure that I did somehow."

She laughed and said, "It didn't really slow me down much. It just made me fatter. I had a boot, and after a month they put a cast on because, of course, I just never slowed down with the boot." Karen rolled her eyes and shook her head.

"I'm involved in a big fundraiser every year for the school district. It's for 700 people, and I do all the decorating for it and the tables. It's a huge space—they tent a tennis court—and you need huge props. I've gotten people from Sony Pictures to help with the props. It's a fabulous affair. I think I was trying to be a superhero: I'm not going to let anything stop me. Nobody's going to say that cancer got the better of me. Oh, it was *terrible*. I was *stupid*." She shook her head disgustedly.

"I almost ended up in the hospital. My white blood count was low, and I was working myself to the bone. I think it was a coping mechanism. My parents were dying. I had the cancer. My foot was broken. I think I was trying to run ahead of this … Take, for instance, doing training walks for the 3-Day. The reason I didn't train adequately was because I don't have enough hours in the day. That's ridiculous because this is my health. First of all, it's not healthy to be 50 pounds overweight—it doesn't make walking any easier—plus, it's not wise to not take care of your health."

In retrospect, Karen understood that nurturing others at the expense of taking care of herself, coupled with reluctance to insist on further diagnostic studies, may have delayed her diagnosis of breast cancer by two years. "When I felt something in my breast, I was probably about 45 or 46. I'd had a mammogram in May of 1999, and I actually went to the doctor and said, 'I feel something in my breast. I don't know what it is, and I don't know if it's anything to worry about, but I feel something.'

"To me, it felt like a thickening rather than a mass. It wasn't anything you could get your fingers around. It just felt different. In fact, it bothered me so much that I would check it all the time—pushing on it. I called the doctor and made an appointment and told her I had a concern, that I had felt a difference. She, of course, did a breast exam, and said that she didn't think it was anything—that what I was feeling was the breast bone. They did a mammogram and, of course, the mammogram didn't show anything. I was just so happy because I didn't want to believe it was anything.

"I continued to feel the thickening. It never got bigger; it never changed, but it always bothered me a little. Still, I figured I must be fine since the mammogram was negative and my doctor wasn't concerned. I missed my mammogram in May of 2000, and so I didn't ..." Karen's voice trailed off, and she walked in silence for a few moments before continuing.

"Anyway, in December of 2001, I was lying on my bed, on my chest, and I felt like I was lying on a rock. That is when I thought, This is not right. Something's wrong. I couldn't tell exactly where it was because, when I stood up, I couldn't palpate anything, but when I lay on it, it felt like it was very deep in there. When I looked in the mirror, from a profile, there was a rippling of the skin of that breast—not the nipple, just the breast itself. When the weight of the breast brought it down, you could see that it was retracted.

"I called my own doctor—it was right at Christmas time, 2001. I had had a mammogram and a doctor's appointment scheduled for January [2002], but I called in December to say that I had felt something and asked if I could please come in earlier. They basically said, 'You have an appointment scheduled for January, so let's just leave it for then. We just don't have time.' People were sick, I guess. It was the holidays." Karen shrugged.

"So I went to see another doctor, just to get some reassurance. That doctor said that she felt what I was feeling and thought that it was probably hormonal, but she recommended a diagnostic mammogram. When I called back my regular doctor and told her—I didn't know the difference between a regular mammogram and a diagnostic mammogram—that I had a prescription for a diagnostic mammogram, her office staff told me, 'Go get it with that doctor because she's the one that wrote you the prescription.'

"I said, 'But you're my doctor, and I've had all my mammograms through Cedars-Sinai, and I want to do it there. Could I please get a diagnostic one?' They said, 'Yes,' and that's when it all started.

"January 29 [2002] was my mammogram. It's funny how you remember those dates." Karen grinned and shook her head. "They did a mammogram. They did a second mammogram, and I thought, Oh dear. Then they came in and said, 'We're going to do an ultrasound. We can see a little area that is of concern.' I said, 'Well, do you see something?' They're so sweet, you know, so they said, 'We just want to check out something.'

"They did the ultrasound and, because it was a diagnostic mammogram, the radiologist read it immediately and called me into the x-ray room and said that she saw a mass; that it was not a cyst; that it was a high probability that it was cancer. She showed it to me. It was kind of like pulling in on itself."

I said, "Like a starburst?"

Karen said, "Exactly! Like a starburst. She said that I needed to see a doctor immediately; that this was serious. I remember leaving her office and calling my husband and just crying, saying, 'Omigod. Omigod.'

"I remember, he said, 'Oh, Karen, you must have heard it wrong. They wouldn't be able to tell that it's cancer by an x-ray. They have to do a biopsy. How would they possibly know?' But I remember saying, 'She knew. She sees thousands of mammograms, and she wouldn't have said what she did unless she was convinced that it was a malignancy.'

"I would do my yearly physical and mammogram on the same day, so I went right from my mammogram to my doctor's office. She basically said, 'I am so sorry.' I mean, what *would* she say?" Karen cocked her head, raised her eyebrows, and looked at me over her sunglasses. "I was pretty resentful. I felt like in May of '99—you want to blame someone for why this has happened—she should have ordered a diagnostic mammogram based on what *I* was feeling. In my mind, I felt like maybe it would have shown up, but who knows.

"She offered to make some referrals, but I said, 'No, I need to go. I need to leave.' I just didn't want to use her as a doctor anymore. I felt like she had really let me down … The surgeons believed that I had had it at least five years, based on the type of cells and the size. It was lobular cancer, 3 cm … It was right on the breast bone, exactly where I had always felt it … Two years is a long time in the course of a cancer, I would think. I just felt that it might have shown up if they had done a sonogram two years earlier." Karen pressed her lips together and shook her head.

"I left her office and called a friend of mine, who's a nurse and whose husband is a doctor, and I said, 'What do I do?' Within two days, they had an appointment for me with one of the top surgeons in Los Angeles. My mammogram was on Tuesday; my appointment with the surgeon was on Thursday; I had my surgery on Monday. It was very quick. Another friend of mine had been diagnosed five years prior to me with breast cancer, and I called her, and she recommended her oncologist. I felt like I got together a good team of doctors very quickly.

"For me, it was very important to know that I had good doctors. My anxiety level would increase dramatically when I had to consider treatment choices. People said, 'Get on the Internet and do your research.' In theory, it sounded wonderful but, in reality, it increased my anxiety horribly. People gave me books to read, and *that* increased my anxiety. *Everything* increased my anxiety."

Karen hunched her shoulders, cupped her ears, squeezed her eyes shut, and laughed at herself. "It was better, at that moment, just putting my life in the hands of other people … I didn't give myself time to think or process. I just wanted it out.

"They did the surgery—it was a big lumpectomy—and they thought they had gotten the cancer, and they did a sentinel node biopsy. So that was on Monday. On Tuesday, I developed a huge hematoma in that breast from the surgery, so I went back to the doctor. By then, they had gotten back the results of the sentinel node biopsy, which showed that there was cancer in the sentinel lymph nodes. They scheduled surgery for Wednesday, and they went back in and took all the rest of the nodes.

"In the first surgery, when they took the sentinel node, they actually took three nodes, because there were two that were very close to the sentinel node … All three of those nodes were positive, and there was an additional positive node when they took the rest. They took 14 nodes total … When she removed the hematoma, she ended up taking more breast tissue, because she felt like she hadn't gotten clear margins. In addition to the lobular cancer [found in the initial biopsy material and lumpectomy], she found a bit of ductal cancer, so she was glad that she'd gone back to remove that hematoma. The ductal cancer was a surprise finding."

In contrast to ductal carcinoma, which begins in the ducts that channel milk to the nipple, lobular carcinoma arises from the milk-producing glands—schematically, think brocolli stalk vs. flowerets. Invasive lobular carcinoma is considerably less common than invasive ductal carcinoma, but patients are treated similarly and have a similar outcome. Karen's experience brings up two additional features of lobular cancer. First, it can occur alongside ductal cancer (a mixed pattern); second, it can be more difficult to palpate and to detect on mammogram. A third feature of lobular carcinoma is its greater tendency to be bilateral than ductal carcinoma. So far, so good, with Karen on this last one.

She continued. "I said to my oncologist, 'Look, I'm very strong. I've never been sick a day in my life. I can do this. You just give it to me.' So I had 12 rounds of chemotherapy. It was a lot. I had four cycles of Adriamycin®, which was every three weeks, and then I did eight cycles of CMF—cyclophosphamide, methotrexate, and fluorouracil—every two weeks. The last month, I did it simultaneously with radiation ... For radiation treatment, they did the clavicle, the breast, the axilla. Then I started tamoxifen.

"My oncologist said that, based on studies that she'd seen, the patients who responded well to this treatment had a good 20-year survival rate. She said that the studies haven't gone beyond that ... At the time, I was 47, and I thought, 20 years, that would be 67. To me, you're still in your prime at 67. I want to live *way* longer than that. Having been diagnosed with cancer, I would like to think that I'm cured, but I know that breast cancer is a chronic disease, and that you're never really cured. When that bit of anxiety sets in, I think, Well, if I'm not cured, I'm buying time. There's so much research being done. I can do this. I can handle whatever they have to throw at me. I'll do it."

Those were fierce words—essentially a c'mon-over-here-and-gimme-your-best-shot attitude. Had I not eventually learned the rest of Karen's breast cancer story, I might have been tempted to think that she was running a bluff, particularly in view of her personality. Far from fierce, hers was a gentle, nurturing demeanor, and she found kind things to say about people and to people. In fact, she paid me a compliment that brought tears to my eyes. "You have such a wonderful, loving personality," she said. "I don't know if you know that about yourself. If it weren't heartfelt, you couldn't wheedle anything out of anybody, but you're very easy to talk to, very warm and southern."

Karen was a psychologist, and I considered her opinion about the way I interacted with others akin to a professional assessment. I felt like I'd just been given an A+!

About her job, she said, "I love what I do. I work for the school district and have a very unusual job. I work as part of a multidisciplinary team with very young children who have been identified at birth or up to three years old as not developing typically. I work with a language therapist, an occupational therapist, and a physical therapist. We figure out what's wrong, what's happening. We are the deliverers of the bad news, but the good part is that there's help. Especially at that age, if you intervene early enough, the prognosis is so good, even for kids with severe handicaps or who are autistic.

"I work hard and I work a lot at home. I have less time for the people I love because I work. I probably don't have to work, but it seems to balance me, and it gives me a lot of self-esteem. If I took that away, I don't know if I would be able to fill the time with something that I love as much."

She continued to work throughout her 12 cycles of chemotherapy, and she also continued to take care of her semi-invalid parents. "When I was diagnosed in February [2001], I was caregiving for my parents, who were very ill. My mother had Alzheimer's. She was 85 and needed significant care, and my father was 89 and had severe heart disease. He was to the point where he was in a wheelchair because he'd fallen and broken his hip. I never told my parents that I had breast cancer because I was their primary caregiver. By that point, I had a caregiver who kind of lived with them, but I still went to see them every day, and I couldn't break their hearts. I wore a wig. I got a great wig. I spent a lot of money on it—it was real hair. I felt like I needed to do that so my mother wouldn't know.

"Even though she had Alzheimer's, she would still evaluate me, just like she had evaluated me my whole life. 'Oh, you lost a little weight. You look good,' or 'I don't like that color on you.' She was so cute. So I wore this wig. At first, I had this cheap wig that wasn't very nice, so I wore it with a baseball cap, but my mom didn't like that because she was really a lady and she didn't like baseball caps. She'd say, 'Take that cap off,' and I'd say, 'Oh, Mom, just leave me alone. I've been working out.'

"In fact, when I had surgery on that Monday and developed the hematoma, that breast was enormous, so I stuffed the other side so that when I went over to her house, she wouldn't notice that I was lopsided. Even my good wig bothered her. She'd say, 'I don't think I like the color of your hair,' and I'd say, 'Oh, Mom, the color's fine. I'm just trying new things.' 'Well, I like it curly better than straight.' I'd say, 'Well, you know, I just want straight hair so badly that I'm gonna try straight for a little while.' When I'd kiss her hello, I'd grab both her hands so that she wouldn't try to reach for my hair." Karen smiled slowly and shook her head.

"They never knew. My cousins who knew were sworn to absolute secrecy not to tell their parents. There wasn't anybody over the age of 55 in my family who knew that I had breast cancer because I just couldn't be sure that they wouldn't slip and tell my parents. You know older people." Karen shrugged, and added, "They can't help it. They forget.

"I was so determined that they would die without knowing their daughter had cancer. That would have been the worst thing in the world. They could offer no support to me in any way, so there was absolutely no purpose in telling them. My father was so able-minded, even though he was 89, and it would have absolutely devastated him. I was the apple of his eye. Even though my mother had Alzheimer's, she would have dwelled on it. It would have been like an octopus that had all these legs that didn't have any purpose.

"So that was in February. In May, my mother was diagnosed with pulmonary fibrosis, and she died the day before Mother's Day. I was still in treatment. I'd go to chemo, and then I'd go from chemo to the hospital. When my mom died—I'll cry when I say this, forgive me. I'll never forget it. She took one of my hands, and she said to me, 'Take care of yourself, and be the best person that you can be. You're my angel.' I really had a sense that she kind of knew, but I was still glad that I hadn't told her. I've never regretted that one."

Karen pressed her lips together and walked in silence for a few minutes. She cleared her throat before continuing. "I would never, in a million years, have ever imagined that my mother would die first because my father had been so frail for so many years. They had been together for 72 years, and I don't know which was worse: my mother dying or seeing my father living without her. He made it for four months, and he died right at the end of my treatment. The good side, I think, was that I could absolutely not focus on my cancer. I needed to just be there for them. I just couldn't abandon them."

When I expressed amazement at her strength at making it through such a tough year, she said, "It was terrible, but it gets worse, a little worse. The good and the bad is that I had never had a year like that. I'm one of those people who has been blessed with an incredibly wonderful life. Great family. Great husband. You know how some people seem to have a black cloud that follows them? That was never me. I never had a black cloud, but six weeks after my dad died, Stu [her husband] had a five-way heart bypass." Karen took a deep breath and let it out slowly. "Actually, it was a coupon scan that saved my husband's life. I remember the doctor coming out to me and saying, 'Karen, I know you've had a horrible year with so much loss, but I really have bad news for you. Your husband needs a bypass, and he needs it immediately.'

"I said to him, 'Can we go home and pick a doctor?'" Karen looked over her sunglasses at me again and said, "I mean, you don't look at that lightly, right? Anyway, I remember that the doctor said to me, 'You're going to have to trust me. He's so at risk right now; he's a walking time bomb. He could make it another day, a week, a month. He's got a 95% occlusion at the top—the origin—of all three main arteries, and two of those arteries are blocked in places below the origin." It was a nine-hour surgery, but he's done great. God was there with us for that one."

When asked how her children fared during what, by anyone's standards, was a bad year, she said, "People would say, 'Omigod, those poor children. They lost both their grandparents, and both their parents had life-threatening illnesses.' Adam was 9 and Sean was 15, and they were just unbelievable ... Sean, my older son, was very anxious about me losing my hair. It was very frightening to him that I had to have chemotherapy ... We told him that I had been diagnosed with cancer, and that I was going to opt for chemotherapy as an insurance policy. 'If the price you pay is to have no hair, it is worth it to have that insurance policy,' we told him.

"We were talking to him about cancer and all its implications as though he were an adult. In return, we allowed him to be an adult, as far as asking any questions, at any time. We told him that we would always tell him the truth, that we wouldn't shade it or pad it, and that if he asked us, we would tell him everything we knew, and he could trust us. And, you know, it was great. He seemed to handle it well. The hair loss ..." Karen paused and laughed. "*That* was his greatest fear.

"At 14, 15, it's all about how you look. He was afraid that I would be bald and unattractive and look sick, and his friends would tease him. So I took control of my hair. My doctors told me that I would lose my hair about the 16th or 18th day. I would have these little hair tests, and I would kind of pull on it, and as soon as I was able to pull out five or six strands, I knew I was days away, so I had a head-shaving party. My friends shaved my head. I think it was harder for them than it was for me."

Karen laughed, but then became serious again. "In general, it was the hardest weekend of that entire year—the weekend that I lost my hair. Once I shaved it, I was fine and I felt liberated, but the fear of it coming out was scary for me. I didn't want it to happen to me; I wanted to be in control of that. First, I cut it very, very short, and then on the 15th day, we took it all off.

"I showed my kids, and I showed my husband, and they were okay with it. I put on a hat and told my oldest son to get in the car. He asked, 'Where are we going?' and I said, 'We're going to go around the neighborhood, and we're going to show all your friends.' He got in the car and we went to maybe five or six houses. I took my hat off and I said, 'Okay, guys, what do you think?' and they said, 'Cool. You look pretty cool.' And I said, 'Okay, son. See, I'm cool.'

"With Adam, it didn't go as well initially because he was only eight at the time, and I wanted to give him only as much information as I thought he needed. I told him I had gone to the doctor, and they had done a test, and they found something in my breast. It was like a little pebble, and they were going to take it out, and I was going to have some medicine, and the medicine was going to make my hair fall out, because that was what this particular medicine did, but I was going to be fine. That's what I told him, and I really thought that it was enough information.

"Then I went in to have my surgery, and while I was in—I spent the night in the hospital—I got a call from one of the parents—and I'm so grateful to her, to this day, because she wasn't a close friend, but her son and my son were in the same class—and she said that she just called to see how I was doing. Then she said, 'I hope this isn't inappropriate, but would you mind telling me what you have shared with Adam, because I'm really worried that parents are talking at school, and I'm worried that he's going to overhear something, and I don't know what he knows.'

"When I got home the next day, we brought Adam in and, in very simple terms that he could understand, we said, 'Do you remember that little pebble that we talked about? That little pebble was *cancer*.' We explained it very simply. We said, 'When you hear that word—*cancer*— we don't want you to be frightened. There are people who have very bad cancers, and they can die, but my cancer is a good kind.'

"Just recently, he said, 'Mom, did you have a good cancer or a bad cancer?' I said, 'I had a good cancer,' and he said, 'That's good, because, you know, people die of cancer.'" Karen smiled lovingly. "I said, 'I know, but I'm going to be fine.' Now, he's 11, and he's cognitively able to have a sense of this. At eight, he didn't have that."

Karen realized cancer's potential to isolate her family, so she pre-empted that problem by being frank with others. "I decided immediately that I needed to let everyone know. First, I really believe in the power of prayer. I'm not really a religious person, as far as going to temple every Sabbath, but I really believe the more people who are pulling for you, the better it is. My name was on every church prayer list, every different religion. I had the Catholics; I had the Jews; I had the Christians; I had the Buddhists; I had them all pulling for me.

"The other reason was that I didn't want people to be talking *about* me; I wanted people to be talking *with* me. I had kids who were very active in sports at school. Every weekend, we'd be at some sporting event, and I didn't want to walk into a gym and have everyone whispering, 'There's Karen. She doesn't look so good. She's got *cancer*.'" Karen hunched her shoulders and put her index finger to her lips, pretending to shush someone. "I figured if they all knew, then they didn't have to be whispering. They could just come up to me and say, 'How are you feeling? How's it going? Can I help? What can I do?'"

Her need to feel connected to people also influenced her approach to chemotherapy. "The first time I went to chemo, there were these two people [in the chemotherapy suite]. One woman never even looked up and acknowledged that a new person had come in. Another person was in there with her husband. He was working on his laptop, and she never acknowledged me either. I said to the nurse, 'This isn't going to work for me. I either need to bring people with me, or you need to put me in a room where I can have a gathering.' Part of me was kidding, but part of me was saying, 'I don't want to come here every two or three weeks and look at people who are giving up on life.'

"I didn't want to feel isolated, so I just brought a group. Every chemo treatment, I'd bring an entourage of people because I had this metaphor—this whole visualization— that there were these two armies, and they were going to war. My army was going to win ... We laughed. We had fun. I got so much strength from them because it made me feel like I had to be all the stronger—like I got lots of acknowledgement for being strong ... I'm such a verbal person. I love to talk. I love to tell stories. I think if I were to be given a punishment, it would be to go live in a seminary for a month. Send me to prison." Karen grinned and added, "At least in prison, you get to have breakfast with everyone and talk. I would love it."

After the center-stage immediacy of chemotherapy was past, *and* she no longer had to be strong for her parents, *and* she no longer feared for her husband's life, Karen developed a fear of recurrence. "I think I put everything on hold because of my parents ... When they died, I had grieved the loss of the parents as I knew them for several years. They had no quality of life. My mother lived in a constant state of anxiety and fear and paranoia with her Alzheimer's. Even when my mother was alive, my father lived in a state of sadness for the loss of this woman whom he absolutely adored and the deterioration of his own health. He was so proud. He was in diapers. He was in a wheelchair. Yet, he really was going to meet his commitment to be with her until the end of her life. Once that was accomplished, he was ready. So I don't think I needed to work as much on grieving for them as I needed to work on grieving my own cancer diagnosis ... I remember telling my oncologist, 'I'll be fine because I can't go there.' But, when I finally allowed myself to go there, I got terribly anxious."

Karen's anxiety about recurrence seduced her into demanding a PET [positron emission tomography] scan, despite her oncologist's warning about the potential for a spurious finding. As bad luck would have it, the PET scan showed an ill-defined lung nodule. This finding necessitated a CAT [computerized axial tomography] scan, which proved that the nodule was, indeed, a false positive; however, a liver abnormality was identified by the CAT scan, which, of course, led to a liver scan. The liver scan indicated that the liver abnormality was a hemangioma, which is a benign, usually clinically insignificant, growth of blood vessels. This pinball series of studies took place over about three months and were, despite being standard of care, ultimately pointless. Karen said that the anxiety experienced while waiting for each set of results felt, in retrospect, almost punitive.

"After this, the oncologist said, 'There's a normal amount of anxiety that people feel. There is a fear of recurrence, but most people can manage it. It comes up, you deal with it, you put it in an appropriate place, then you go on with your life. You seem to be worrying about it more than I think is healthy. I think that you might think about going to somebody to talk about it. I think that you're just now grasping that you have cancer. It took two years to get through your parents' dying and your husband's surgery.'

"I actually did make an appointment with a psychologist. I sat down with her and she said, 'Karen, you had a horrible year, and you probably weren't able to process all of that year because it was a horrible year, and nobody could process it.' As I was listening to myself tell her about that year, I thought, Omigod, Karen, get over it. Not get over the year; get over needing to go sit and pay someone to reinvent your life ... And I've actually felt much better since then. I think I needed somebody—some professional person—to tell me that it was a horrible year."

Another way that Karen grappled with fear of recurrence was to attend a three-day retreat for cancer survivors called Healing Odyssey, which is based in Laguna Hills, California, south of Los Angeles. According to the Web site (www.healingodyssey.org), "In 1993, oncology professionals Nancy Raymon, R.N., M.N., A.O.C.N., an oncology nurse specialist, and Donna Farris, L.C.S.W., a clinical social worker, envisioned a three-day cancer survivor support program that would move women quickly and powerfully beyond their cancer experience and back into living well after cancer."

Karen said, "They give you a lot of tools to move beyond fear. It's not like at summer camp where you just go do fun things. There was a lot of processing that was necessary before you could do these activities, and a lot of trust was required. During one activity, you're harnessed to a tree near a boulder that hangs out over a 100-foot canyon drop. I don't know if it was a *hundred* feet, but it looked like the Grand Canyon to me." Karen laughed and continued. "You had to go to the edge of the rock and fall forward. Your feet never left the ground, but your body fell forward until the harness caught you. I did it, and I screamed for about a second or 10 seconds—I don't know how long—because I didn't know if the harness was going to catch me. I mean, *intellectually*, I knew.

"In another rope activity, there were two telephone poles with a beam between them that was 30 feet above the ground. First, you had to climb up the ladder. For some women, that was the challenge—climbing the ladder. After you climbed up the ladder, you had to step onto the supporting beam and let go of the tree, and you had to move across the beam, balancing yourself. Again, you were in a harness that was cabled to a tree and another tree and to six women who were at the end of that rope. Once you got as far as you could go, you fell backwards into the air, and the cable caught you, and the women basically caught you and lowered you down." Karen hunched her shoulders and shuddered.

"It involved incredible trust ... It was an amazingly powerful exercise about moving beyond fear. I remember being up on that beam. My knees were shaking and I was so afraid. I kind of like being high, but I'd never been that high. It was such a clarifying moment in my life because I thought to myself, Just get focused, Karen. Just put the things in front of you that mean so much to you, and keep looking beyond the treetops. I thought, Just keep looking out there and keep moving across that beam. If you put what's important in front of you, you can do this. I did it. I was one of the few who made it across the beam, and it really taught me the importance of being in the present. I'm always looking forward to the next day instead of enjoying the present one. I needed to learn that lesson, and it's been a hard lesson for me."

Toward the end of the route on Day 1, a member of the Warming Hut Hotties team caught up with Karen and me. She was friendly and funny, and she gave us stickers that said "Honorary Hottie." The Warming Hut Hotties were the largest team at the San Francisco 3-Day, with 120 members, and they raised over $330,000. Its members were easy to spot because they all wore plastic head bands with springy antennae, which were topped with pink, fuzzy balls. When the Hotties walked, their antennae jiggled.

Since our Hottie walking buddy was obviously familiar with the area, Karen and I asked where, exactly, we were. She pointed out the bridge that connects San Mateo and San Francisco Bay. She pointed towards Oakland and Berkeley and told us that the Golden Gate Bridge would be behind a little mound of trees, there in the distance. Then she said, "See that little crop of trees right there? That's where we will be camping tonight."

I said, "Oh, yeah, I see it. Is that a little peninsula?"

The Warming Hut Hottie said, "Uh huh. That's called Coyote Point."

"*Coyote* Point? Why is it called that?"

The Hottie cocked her head, which made her antennae jiggle even more than usual, grinned at me, and said, "I don't know. Maybe there are some coyotes there." She shrugged and added, "That would make sense, don't you think?"

She was obviously enjoying herself, so I didn't answer. Instead, I was thinking about camping in a place called Coyote Point. My peripheral vision was already sharpening.

In contrast to Karen Schweibish, breast cancer survivor, Cathy Schwandt, 52, never gave recurrence a passing thought. She said there were two reasons for this. First, she survived a childhood illness that was supposedly fatal. ("They told my parents that I was going to die by the time I was six.") Second, she was diagnosed with breast cancer at an early age. ("I was 28 years old and invincible and immortal and had the attitude of 'Just take it out and let's be done with it.'")

About the childhood illness, she said, "When I was two, I woke up one morning with juvenile rheumatoid arthritis. I had a big swollen knee. My parents—I was born in Michigan—took me to the hospital and the doctor diagnosed it as water on the knee. At two years old, they diagnosed it as *water on the knee.*" Cathy shook her head, harrumphed, and continued. "Somewhere along the line, the doctor diagnosed it as juvenile rheumatoid arthritis. I was in the hospital 13 times by the time I was seven. I didn't know until much later that I was supposed to die by the time I was six ... Having been sick as a child, I thought that breast cancer was just another thing. My attitude was like, Okay, make it go away like everything else that has gone away in my life.

"I did the regular OB/GYN pap yearly thing and he found a lump. Back then, in 1981, you didn't hear about breast self-exams or breast cancer. It was kind of hush-hush. So he said, 'Go to this doctor down the hall.' I couldn't tell you now, but I think he must have been a surgeon ... So I went down the hall, and the guy said, 'Oh, yeah. We need to do a biopsy.' So I went to the hospital—it was here in San Francisco—but I didn't tell my family. My best friend took me. The surgeon said, 'We need to go in, and if it's malignant, we'll need to do a mastectomy,' and I said, 'Okay, but how will I know?' He said, 'Well, if you wake up and have to stay, it's malignant, but otherwise you can just go home afterwards.'

"I went in—my friend took me, I wasn't married at the time—and I woke up in the Recovery Room, and the first thing out of my mouth was, 'Do I have to stay here?' and they said, 'Yes.' I was still kind of foggy, but I said, 'Okay, but I need to tell my friend.' The next thing I remember is that I'm in my room, checked in, and I'm still trying to comprehend what is going on, and my sister, Pat, shows up at my bedside. Pat's here. She's the one, back there, who brought me Starbuck's."

Cathy paused to take a gulp from the latte that her sister had brought for her. "Mmmm. Anyway, Pat shows up at my bedside. Nobody in my family knew that I was going to be there, so I said, 'How did you know that I was here?' and she said, 'Well, I called work, and they said you had a doctor's appointment, so I called our doctor'—we went to the same doctor—'and they said that you weren't there, but to try Dr. G.'s office. I called there, and they told me that you had just had a biopsy and had been diagnosed with breast cancer, and had been admitted to the hospital.'

"They didn't know if that was my sister. It could have been anybody. So that's how she found out. She lives in Pacifica, so it was close, and she was just like ..." Cathy paused and made a quick, swooping motion with her hand, "... *there*. She called my other sister, who lives in the East Bay, and they got on the phone to the American Cancer Society. At the time, that was the only support group available. They told us to get a second opinion and gave us some doctors' names. We told Dr. G. that we wanted a second opinion, and he brought in a second doctor who said, 'Yeah, you need to have a radical mastectomy.'

"My sister said, 'Well, how does he know? He's the guy that operated on my *knee*.' He didn't check me or anything." Cathy squinted her eyes and, with her voice higher pitched than before and reflecting righteous indignation, added, "*I was 28 ... years ... old ... and an orthopedic surgeon was saying that I needed a radical mastectomy ... without ... even ... checking ... me!*" When she saw my jaw drop, she said, "Unbelievable, right?"

Cathy's voice returned to normal, and she continued. "My sister said, 'You're not staying here. We're going to go talk to one of these other doctors on the list.' So we called and made appointments, and I ended up going to a surgeon, Dr. Richards—he might be dead now because he was old then—and he said that he needed the biopsy report and the mammogram. Trying to get those was almost impossible. They didn't want to give them to me. We did get them, but it took us a couple of weeks. Meanwhile, I had to call my parents, who lived in southern California, and they came up.

"I only wish I could remember the name of the oncologist at UC [the University of California in] San Francisco, because he was wonderful. My mother and I had a major consultation with him, and he explained all the options to me. The surgeon, Dr. Richards, had already told me a couple of different things, but he had said, 'I want you to go talk to him [the oncologist] and find out about everything.' So I talked to the oncologist, and he said, 'You can have a radical mastectomy and be done with it; or, based on its size and where it is, you can have a modified radical mastectomy, where we take out only some of the muscle that runs behind the breast and the lymph nodes; or you can take out the lump and the lymph nodes and, if there's nothing in the lymph nodes, we can just keep an eye on it.' Based on what I've learned since, I've realize how cutting edge that last option was. Like I said, I wish I could remember his name."

Actually, Cathy's surgeon *was* on the cutting edge. In 1981, when she was diagnosed, modified radical mastectomy was still considered the ideal surgical treatment for breast cancer. In fact, in 1981, it had only been a little over a decade since modified radical mastectomy had replaced radical mastectomy as the standard of care. As functionally and cosmetically unacceptable as it was, the radical mastectomy, developed by William Halstead, M.D., in 1893, was still superior to breast amputation, which, prior to 1846, when general anesthesia was developed, was done as rapidly as possible with women awake. As would be expected, the fatality rate was very high from the surgical procedure—if you can even call it that—or from subsequent infection.

Cathy continued. "I went back to Dr. Richards and told him what I wanted to do. They called it a partial mastectomy. I think, these days, it would be the same thing as a lumpectomy or a wide local excision. At any rate, they took out the lump and the lymph nodes. I'm kind of caved in right here." She looked down and patted the outer aspect of her left breast. "I never knew what kind of cancer it was. It was so long ago, and back then, I didn't know what they were talking about. I was like, 'Just take it out, and tell me I'm fine, and let me go away ...' I was in the hospital for about five or six days. They took out all of the lymph nodes, and they tested them, and they were all clear. They told me that it was as big as a walnut, which I found out later is pretty big. I didn't do chemo. I didn't do radiation. I said, 'No,' to all that. They gave me the odds—the percentages—I can't tell you what they told me—but, obviously, I felt comfortable with deciding that I didn't want to do any of that stuff.

"They said that they'd just keep checking me, and I said, 'Okay.' Of course, back then, I smoked and took birth control pills. I stopped the birth control pills. That was the one thing that they told me I couldn't do anymore. They didn't know if that was a cause, but they said not to take them anymore, so I said, 'Okay.' I just kept going back. First, it was every three months for a mammogram—that was for a year. And then it went to six months, and that was probably for about five years, and then it was yearly. They never talked about breast self-exams. I never heard about that until much, much later.

"The only thing that bothered me was that I lost some mobility in my arm for a while. They showed me exercises to walk my arm up the side of the wall and that kind of thing. When I played softball, I'd reach for a ball and my arm wouldn't go. It kind of stuck there. To this day, I'm still numb in a certain part. Other than that, I never really thought about it again. It just wasn't an issue." Cathy shrugged.

When asked if she ever talked to anyone about breast cancer, she said, "There was this one lady at work who had breast cancer, but she was very, very ill, and she eventually died. I probably was the last person she needed to talk to, being this young kid. She was a really nice lady, I remember, with young kids. Even that didn't connect in my brain, because she was older, and I really felt this kind of immortality at 28."

Over the years, though, as she met other breast cancer survivors and listened to their stories, Cathy gained insight into the bullet that she had dodged. Interestingly, as she learned more about breast cancer treatment and survivorship, her youthful insouciance was not replaced by gratitude, but by guilt. She became tearful when she tried to describe her reasons for feeling this way. "I felt guilty after meeting people and reading stories and hearing people talk about chemo and seeing them lose their hair and everything else. I thought, I never suffered like that. I don't have the *right* to say that I'm a survivor, because I never suffered. I just treated it so trivially. Twenty-four years of survival without medications or anything ..." Cathy's voice trailed off.

She paused to wipe away tears before continuing. "I felt like I hadn't *earned* the right to wear a pink shirt. I felt like I had cheated ... I'm doing better now, the more I do events like the 3-Day, and the more I talk to people, but that has been a major thing that I never told people about.

"There's another thing that happened that eased a little bit of the guilt. About a year and a half ago, I had a mammogram and they saw calcifications. They were looking at these little pinprick things, and I was saying, 'I don't see them,' and they said, 'Yeah, they're there.' I said, 'Whatever.' So they said, 'We'll watch it. Come back in six months,' and I said, 'Okay.' It was probably a year later that the radiologist said, 'I think I want to biopsy this.' When he told me that, my reaction was, 'Wait a minute. I'm not invincible,' but then I thought, 'Cathy, don't worry about it. There's nothing you can do about it until you know what it is, so don't even lose sleep over this. It's probably nothing.' And it wasn't anything—just some scar tissue—but I have to say that there was a little twinge of concern for a while. I look back now and wonder how I could have been so flippant for so long over something so serious."

Still, though, as part of the effort to sort out her feelings about being a long-time survivor, she became involved in Race for the Cure® and long-distance walks. Her first 3-Day was in San Francisco in 2001. The following year, she walked in Washington, D.C., and in 2003, she crewed for an Avon 2-Day. Michigan's first 3-Day event was held in 2002, and that was the year that Cathy Schwandt became Dancing Lady.

"Dancing Lady really derived from Pretty Woman Man. When I did San Francisco the first time, I remember how great it was to come across him playing *Pretty Woman*." (She was referring to a man who drove a van along the route, playing Roy Orbison's *Pretty Woman* over a loud-speaker.) "It would make you pick up your step a little bit. When the first Michigan 3-Day event came about, I thought, They don't know anything about the 3-Day walk up there. They don't know what it's about, and nobody up there will know to do something like that, so I decided to go up and play music.

"I put together a CD of different songs, all kind of disco-ish. It ended up, when I was playing the music for everyone and cheering, I started dancing. When I hear music, I dance. I just can't help myself … I got e-mails later saying, 'Thank you,' and 'Are you going to do it again next year?' There were people who said, 'I walked for you,' and 'You were my inspiration,' and 'Dancing Lady, you were awesome.' One said, 'If it weren't for you, I wouldn't have made it the last day.' I would read the e-mails and cry." Her chin quivered and she nodded slowly.

Turning to me, she said, "If I could, I'd do what you do. I would walk them all. I like to talk to people and hear their stories and find out why they're here. That's the true meaning of what this is all about."

———

Another walker who recognized the value of sharing stories was Jerry McCollum, 38, a three-year survivor of myxoid liposarcoma, a highly aggressive malignant tumor that arises in fatty tissue. He said that sharing his cancer story and listening to the stories of the other walkers were healing for him. This was, perhaps, more true for him than for many breast cancer survivors. For one thing, because of its rarity, he has found that few people grasp the meaning of his diagnosis. "When I say myxoid liposarcoma, for all they know, I'm talking about a flower. They have no idea." Furthermore, Jerry said that his wife and other family members choose not to discuss the significance of the lung metastasis that was discovered when he had a follow-up scan.

When we talked about the gravity of metastatic disease, he said, "Do I feel helpless? Sometimes. There's no one to really talk to except for yourself. I feel like I'm going to die from this, but there's not that many people out there who have the knowledge, I guess. But when you talk to a certain group of people who know exactly what it is, they give you a look or a frown, and say, 'Omigod, how'd you get it?'"

Jerry described the events that led to his diagnosis of cancer. "I was getting ready for work, getting dressed, putting on my pants, and the pants leg on my left leg would not go above my calf. I was 35 at the time, three years ago. My wife and I would joke about it, because we thought it was a spider bite, but a week goes by, and it's getting bigger and bigger. We finally decided to see a doctor. There was no pain at all. No redness at all. It was just swollen. When we saw the general doctor, she said that she could guarantee that it was not a spider bite, but that she had no idea what it was.

"After three or four weeks of testing, they came up with exactly what it was. By then, it had started pushing on the nerves in my leg, and my leg had started going numb throughout the day ... The doctor at Kaiser suggested that my leg be amputated ... My wife and I found a guy on the Internet—a surgical oncologist in South San Francisco, Dr. Richard O'Donnell [Chief, Orthopaedic Oncology Service, University of California San Francisco Cancer Center], who e-mailed us back and agreed to meet with us and check it out ... He wasn't with Kaiser, but he agreed to do a limb salvage operation if Kaiser would pay for it; in return, he would show the Kaiser doctors how to do the surgery."

While Jerry was recovering from surgery—before he was even able to bear weight on his leg—he saw a commercial for the 3-Day event and decided that he wanted to participate. He figured that his family would try to discourage him, so he raised the money and began training for the event without telling them. Just six months after his surgery, he walked 60 miles in the San Francisco 3-Day event. In 2003, he walked again, and in 2004, he walked in all three California 3-Day events (San Diego, Los Angeles, and San Francisco). About his first 3-Day event, he said, "During Day 0 and Day 1, I realized that it had nothing to do with me and my leg. It was about the ladies and the amazing stories that you hear out here—the survivors and the ones that have passed ... I met some amazing ladies that listened to me and who shared their stories.

"The hardest part for me is when it's over. You go home, and life is still the same. It's nice walking these three together, because I can see everybody, but after it's over, I feel like, 'Where'd everybody go?'"

Jerry grew up in South Carolina and joined the military right after high school. He served five years in the U.S. Army Infantry and saw combat with the Panamanian defense league during Operation Just Cause. He now works at a forklift company, plays on two softball teams, and volunteers at a children's hospital in Oakland. "Every Wednesday night, I can't think of a better place to go ... I call my little oncology friends my 'mini-me's' ... There are a lot of kids, even now at the hospital, that I can help by sharing my story ... There are times when the kids don't want to get an IV, and I say, 'I know that it hurts, but they only want to make you better. Without certain medicines, you will get worse.' I'll talk to the nursing staff and tell them to give me an IV to show the kids that it's not that bad. Of course, I hate needles more than anybody, but the nurse will start an IV, and I will not flinch or move. They'll even run it through, like a saline solution.

"I've had three angels pass away since I've been volunteering there. All three of them were amazing little ones, and I'm sure they're waiting for the guy in the blue jacket to show up and visit and play with them one day. They're amazing—the kids there. Just amazing."

On Day 3, it started drizzling during breakfast and, by the time the route opened, it was raining hard. I spent most of the morning behind a contingent of the Warming Hut Hotties who, with their drenched puff-balled antennae, looked like a cluster of wet, cheerful cats. Our route departed from camp in South San Francisco and soon passed through Kohlman, with its block after block of cemeteries. The wet cats grew somber as we passed by the thousands of grave sites. Their cheerfulness returned, though, once we returned to the livelier streets of Daly City and St. Francis Wood in San Francisco.

During lunch, I checked my cell phone voicemail and had a message from one of my best friends from San Antonio, René Rone. She and her husband, Fred Lesieur, had hoped to surprise me but, with the sketchy weather, decided that they had better let me know ahead of time that they were planning to meet me at Closing Ceremonies at Golden Gate Park. The message went on to say that if the Golden Gate Park convergence failed, they had reservations at the same hotel where I was staying on Sunday night. I never had any doubt that they would be there, waiting for me, and they were, of course, with roses and hugs and heartfelt job-well-done-Debs. I felt like a returning warrior. It was one of the high points of all the 3-Day events.

Despite the overcast skies and shivery weather, there was only a hint of mist during the first parts of Closing Ceremonies. Three groups were introduced separately as they entered the stage area: the Warming Hut Hotties; the San Jose Police Department; and the Hookers for Hooters, a group of women and cross-dressing men who drove up and down the route in a convertible, playing music, *yoo-hooing*, blowing kisses, and periodically stopping the car to spill out and pose for vaguely lewd photographs with walkers. All three groups received applause but, predictably, the officers of the San Jose Police Department pegged the applause-o-meter.

Since 2000, members of the San Jose Police Department have volunteered to provide safety for breast cancer walks in the San Francisco Bay Area. They also offer "support and encouragement" and, to that end, several officers, wearing their bike shorts, visited Camp One to sell and sign their 2005 calendar, "Why We Ride." All proceeds from calendars were to be "donated towards finding a cure," and sales were brisk.

The calendar photographs featured one or more members of the force, including their reasons for riding. One of my favorite quotes from "Why We Ride" was Sergeant Larry McGrady's: "I ride because of the respect we receive from the walkers. I ride for them, but they support us. We each share, we each give, and we all come together for this great cause." (For edification purposes, Sergeant McGrady was stunningly handsome. That wasn't the reason, though, that his was one of my favorite quotes. Truly, it wasn't. Really.) But back to San Francisco's misty, chilly Closing Ceremonies.

Just as the Survivors' Circle began moving toward the stage, the wind kicked up, and the real rain started—to the squeals of women. In the center of the circle, holding the blue flag, was Brandon Cruz, 16, whose mother, Amelita (Amy) Cruz, had died of breast cancer less than two months before, on August 22, 2004. She was 47. He and his father, Michael, were both walking in the event, and I briefly spoke with Michael on Day 2.

Amy was first diagnosed in February 2001, was treated aggressively, and did well until May 2003, when she was found to have metastatic disease in her liver and bones. Michael said, "They gave her Taxotere® and that seemed to have done a really good job. She was back to work in October [2003]. It was about three months ago that she started experiencing excruciating pain in her hips, and they found that her hips were full of cancer. They tried to treat her, but it was already too far along."

Shortly before she died, Amy was hospitalized, and the attending physician told Michael that his wife would soon pass away. Michael had difficulty maintaining his composure when he told me about his wife's final days. "I had to tell Amy what the doctor told me—that she might not make it past the weekend ... I had to tell the kids that Mommy might not make it past the weekend, and we called my family. My mom and my sister live on Guam—that's where I'm originally from—and they flew out immediately. My sister from Hawaii flew out immediately, as well as her brother from Chicago and his family. Everyone came out. I have relatives that live here, too, and they were all very supportive.

"We did everything. We're Catholic, and we started a healing rosary and prayed and did all that. She made it past the weekend, actually, until the following Sunday, and that's when she passed." We walked without talking for a few minutes.

Michael continued, occasionally pausing to clear his throat. "Someone had told us, just before she passed, that there's a time that you have to let them know that it's okay to go. I was sitting with my daughter—

Jenice, she's 19—and I asked her, 'Did you tell Mommy that it's okay to go?' and she said, 'No, not yet.'

"So I said, 'Okay.' We both got up—my son, Brandon, was on the other side of the bed, and I said, 'Brandon, you need to tell Mommy that it's okay to go,' and he said, 'Yeah, I've been telling her.' So we told her—my daughter and I—and I bent down to kiss her, and that was her last breath. She exhaled right after I kissed her and told her that I loved her. That was pretty hard. When they say to let them know that it's okay to go, I didn't expect her to go that quickly. It was getting close. I thought she was waiting for her best friend, Cathy Kissinger, and her family, but she was waiting for us to tell her it was okay to go. She just exhaled. We called the nurse in, and they pronounced her dead at 5:55 on the 22nd."

Michael bowed his head, drew in a deep breath, and then looked up at the sky. Tears began to trickle down his cheeks. We walked in silence for a while, and then I told him about my husband's final moments and my reaction to his death. It's something that I have only shared with a few people. I can't write about it.

Michael and I talked about the effect of a parent's death on teenage children. "Right now, I think my son is doing the best of the three of us. He's talking to the bereavement counselor at school twice a week. My daughter is still in denial, as I am sometimes, too. I don't believe she's gone sometimes. I expect to come home from a business trip ..." Michael's voice trailed off, and he shook his head.

When he spoke again, his voice was husky. "Brandon went on his own to talk to the counselor at school, which was great. He said, 'Dad, I know I can talk to you, but I'd just like to talk to someone who is detached from the situation and has no emotional ties.' My son surprises me a lot with his maturity. My daughter, at this point, is not ready to talk to a professional. She's still trying to put her arms around it. She actually took this semester off from college, and she's got a part-time job at a restaurant. It's keeping her mind busy and she's keeping active.

"Right now, we're still trying to accept it, but it's going to be a while. We're a close family. Amy and I were married for 21 years." Michael's voice grew husky again, and he swallowed hard. I reiterated what I had told him at the beginning of our conversation—not to feel any pressure to continue talking to me—but he composed himself and said, "I want to talk, because I think it helps me. I want our conversation to be in a book, because when people read what I say, it's going to keep Amy living in their hearts. I want to do that. I want to find ways that I can to do that."

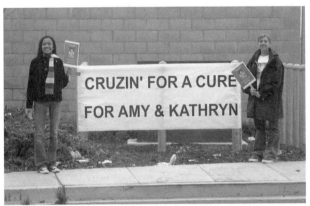

San Francisco boosters

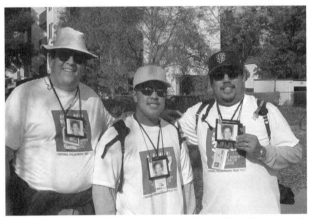

Family members John Rudolph, Brandon Cruz, and Michael Cruz

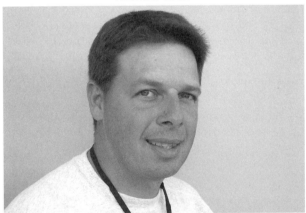

Jerry McCollum

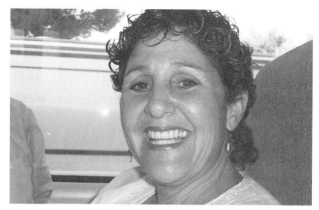

Karen Schweibish

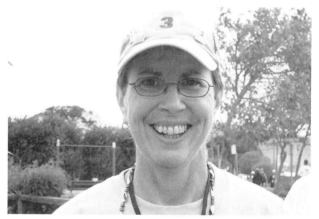

Cathy Schwandt

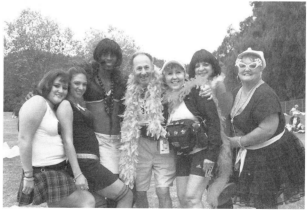

*Bob and Barbara Jo Kirshbaum
with Hookers for Hooters*

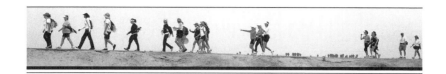

Chapter 10

Arizona
October 22, October 23, and October 24, 2004

On Day 0 of the Arizona 3-Day, while crossing the unpaved parking lot of Scottsdale's Rawhide Western Town on my way to registration, I felt a dusty surge of wind and a single, swift raindrop. I turned to the woman walking beside me and said, "I think we'd better make a run for it." She looked at me like she thought I'd lost my marbles, so I added, "No, really. I know the desert. It's fixing to pour."

I began running toward the Rawhide Pavilion, which was about 50 yards away. As I passed others who were walking, I shouted, "Y'all better hurry." I'm not sure if anyone paid any attention, but there were people ahead of me who had already started to run. I skidded into the Pavilion, out of breath, just as the desert clouds delivered on their promise. Trying my best not to be smug, I thought, Those people who were lollygagging must not have experienced abrupt desert downpours; those of us who were licketysplitting sure had. I later learned that 46 states were represented among the 1,900 walkers and 230 crew members at the Arizona 3-Day. This explained some of the lollygagging.

During the Arizona summer, monsoon thunderstorms originate from southerly and southeasterly winds off the Pacific Ocean and the Gulf of Mexico but, during the winter, winds come from California and Nevada. As predicted in that morning's edition of the *East Valley Tribune*, Arizona's "first winter storm" arrived as we walked (and ran) across the parking lot. Within an hour and a half of the first raindrops, the temperature dropped from 86 to 63 degrees. Later, as I stood in line at the 3-Day store to pay for a warm-up suit, I overheard a woman with a New York-sounding accent say, "What's up with this weather? I thought Arizona was supposed to be hot. You know, tumbleweeds and lizards and that kinda crap."

This woman was obviously unfamiliar with the capriciousness of desert weather, but not me. Our family left West Texas's desert when I was 10 years old, but not before I unwittingly absorbed an understanding of desert weather which, to this day, remains ingrained. Granted, Scottsdale's desert is the Sonoran, with saguaro and senita, and my childhood's desert was the Chihuahuan, with lechuguilla and sotol. Even so, similarities exist.

————

According to Penny Burczyk, 43, of Chandler, Arizona, weather knowledge was not the only thing that people unwittingly absorbed from where they live. She believed that environmental toxins in her native northwest Indiana contributed to the high incidence of cancer among her family and friends, and that, unfortunately, the effects of environmental toxins were not cast off when she left there in 1994 and moved to Arizona.

Certainly, the evidence was compelling: Penny's mother died of breast cancer. One of her older brothers died of liver cancer, and another brother has undergone multiple resections for malignant melanoma. An older sister survived uterine cancer, but later died of colon cancer at age 48. Another older sister was diagnosed with preinvasive uterine cancer in her early 30s, which required a hysterectomy. Her sister-in-law, who grew up in northwest Indiana, had breast cancer. One of her friends, who grew up in Indiana, but who moved to Arizona, was diagnosed with a rare type of lung cancer. This friend's younger sister, who moved to Texas, has undergone bilateral mastectomy for breast cancer. Her childhood best friend's father died from lung cancer in his 40s, and Penny is a survivor of both breast and ovarian cancer.

Although she was warm and friendly to me, I had the sense that, in some settings at least, Penny's natural tendency would be towards shyness. (This is not a criticism. I happen to personally understand that tendency.) Certainly, she was not a foot-stamping, rabble-rousing, hysterical type. However, when describing the staggering amount of cancer among those she loved, she became indignant.

"Something really needs to be done. I say that it's something in the environment because I grew up in northwest Indiana—in a place called The Region—which is very close to a lot of refineries and all the steel mills ... That's where everybody worked when I was little, the steel mills. We all drank the water because we didn't have bottled water ... I've seen articles that say that the cancer rate is higher in these certain regions. Actually, Kelly, my niece, who graduated from IU—Indiana University in Bloomington—double majored in environmental management and public finance and minored in economics, did a research paper on it, and the results were astounding."

Penny's niece investigated the incidence of cancer in northwest Indiana. In other words, she posed the question, "Is there more cancer here than in other places?" The answer appeared to be, "Absolutely." The next question was, of course, "Why is that so?"

Unfortunately, despite exhaustive scientific investigation, the contributing factors (etiology) for most types of cancer are hardly straightforward. Take, for instance, lung cancer, which is caused by cigarette smoking, right? Not necessarily. Thirteen percent of people who die from lung cancer never smoked. Conversely, all of us know someone who smoked two packs a day of unfiltered Lucky Strikes®, lived to 87, raising hell and telling jokes 'til the end, only to topple off their horse while roping an unruly calf—or some variation thereof. Put another way: Cancer etiology is complicated.

Breast cancer's etiology is no exception. In fact, an entire section of every issue of *Breast Diseases: A Year Book® Quarterly* deals with epidemiology and etiology. The physician editors of this excellent publication rifle through over 350 medical and allied health journals and pick out the articles that the rest of us need to know about.

Although recent issues of *Breast Diseases* didn't review any literature concerning specific geographic regions, here were some of the other subjects:

• germline mutations ("… mutations in genes other than *BRCA1* and *BRCA2* are associated with a high risk of breast cancer, particularly in young women")

• induced abortion and miscarriage ("… do not support the hypothesis that induced abortion or miscarriage increases breast cancer risk in young women")

• oral contraceptive use ("… increased risk of lobular carcinoma but not with an increased risk of ductal carcinoma")

• exposure to fertility medications ("… more advanced disease … particularly aggressive … poorer prognosis …")

• diet ("… protective effects of fruits and certain vegetables against breast cancer.")

• smoking ("… may be associated with a small increase in the risk of breast cancer …")

• hormone replacement therapy ("… [users of] combined estrogen and continuous testosterone-like progestins were more than 4 times as likely as never-users to develop breast cancer")

• severe caloric restriction ("… may confer protection against breast cancer)

• weight gain ("… strongly associated with post-menopausal breast cancer only among women who did not use HRT [hormone replacement therapy]")

• dietary phytoestrogens ("… high intake of isoflavones or mammalian lignans was not associated with breast cancer risk.")

• carbohydrate intake ("… risks being greater among women with a BMI [body mass index] of 25 or more.")

• daily aspirin ("… associated with a reduced risk of breast cancer.")

• type 2 diabetes ("… slightly higher risk …")

I could grind on, but the point is that anyone who claims to have a simple answer does not comprehend the complexity of the question. And—indulge me for one paragraph, please—while I'm spouting off about etiology and oversimplification, I would like to go on record as saying that those who criticize the Susan G. Komen Foundation for inadequately funding etiologic studies are off target. The Komen Foundation's scientific advisory board chooses not to fund studies that are underpowered or poorly conceived or redundant or simply not worthwhile. Before I climb down from my high horse, I want to add that I wouldn't walk 600 miles for an organization that doesn't have their ducks in a row when it comes to allocating research funds.

As the accounting supervisor for the City of Chandler, Penny Burczyk is more attuned to responsible spending than most of us. She graduated from Indiana University with a degree in accounting and worked in Indiana until two years after her mother's death from breast cancer. She and her husband, Steve, who is 10 years her senior, then moved to Arizona. Steve is a retired police officer who now works as a security supervisor. After they relocated, she worked for the City of Phoenix, but later accepted her present position in nearby Chandler. She said that she loves her job but admitted that it sometimes entailed extra hours. Her job's demands became a bone of contention after her cancer experiences.

Her breast cancer was discovered on a screening mammogram in December 2002. Penny said, "The funny thing about my lump was that they called me to say, 'We see irregularities; we need you to come in.' I was supposed to go in the next day. That next morning in the shower, my lump popped out, which blew my mind. You definitely notice when a lump on your breast pops out like that. I said, 'Look, Steve, here it is,' and he said, 'Oh, my goodness.'"

The irregularity turned out to be infiltrating carcinoma. She had a lumpectomy and sentinel node biopsy, followed by eight cycles of combination chemotherapy and radiation. "All this time I was still working, except I would schedule my chemo on Fridays, in the afternoon, so that I could get back to work on Mondays. I started that in January [2003], and in April I had a small infection and was hospitalized for a little over a week for a blood transfusion and that type of stuff ... When they were doing some tests in the hospital, they found a cyst on my left ovary.

"After I was discharged, they monitored the cyst with ultrasounds, and it actually kept growing. I only had one more chemo treatment left, so I asked my gynecologist, 'Could you please wait until this last chemo before you do anything?' He said, 'Well, I'm going to send you for another ultrasound. If it gets any bigger, we need to take it out right away.'

"He scheduled the ultrasound a day or two after my last chemo. They called me and said, 'You've got to schedule surgery right away because it has already grown to 10 cm.'

"I had just started a couple of rounds of radiation when I had the ovary removed. It's not a major, major surgery. They made a small bikini cut and did it. I was home recuperating, and my oncologist called me on a Monday and said, 'It appears that your ovary was cancerous as well.'

"Being that I was home recuperating, I was by myself. I said, 'You've got to be kidding me.' He said to make an appointment and to get in right away. I just didn't tolerate it very well." Penny shook her head and added, "Not well at all."

Penny looked away and sighed before continuing. "That was around noontime, and my husband was due to get off work at about two. Steve went with me to the appointment. The medical oncologist told me that the two cancers were not related at all. I asked him what was supposed to happen, and he said he would call me about what to do next. I pressed the issue, and my radiologist, my oncologist, and my gynecologist talked to each other and referred me to a gynecologic oncologist in Phoenix. He told me that there was a 75% chance that cancer was not on my other ovary. I had had a hysterectomy in 2000, but they had left the ovaries. He said, 'We can follow you, or we can go ahead and remove the other ovary. We'll have to remove the lymph nodes. We'll have to remove the omentum [the apron-like fatty deposit that is attached to the large bowel].'

"I said, 'I'm not willing to accept a 25% chance that it's not benign. Let's do the surgery.' I had surgery the day after Labor Day in September of last year [2003] … Everything was okay [no additional tumor was found] but, because it was an aggressive cell type, I had to undergo some more chemo. At that point, I said, 'Okay, we need to put in a portacath.' Even though I had good veins in the beginning, they had problems every darn time they tried to start an IV and had to poke me two, three, four times." Penny pressed her lips together and absentmindedly rubbed her forearm, as if recalling the needle sticks.

She continued. "Of course, they could only work with the left arm. I had the port put in. I started the chemo—Taxol® and cisplatin … I had to wait to start the chemo because I was still doing my radiation, and they were afraid that it would burn me too badly. I was already having problems with burns. I finished radiation in October, started my chemo, then finished that in February of this year [2004].

"They're following me now every four months. I go in for a CAT [computerized axial tomography] scan of my abdomen and pelvis because I have what appear to be cysts on my liver and kidneys, and they want to make sure that those don't grow any. I've had a couple of bone scans. I think one of my biggest fears was that it would go to my bones the way it did with my mother." Penny squinted her eyes and added, "She really suffered with that."

She paused and shook her head before continuing. "Her doctor in Indiana was treating her for leg cramps, but actually the cancer had come back. It wasn't until her regular doctor went on vacation, and she went to the surgeon who had done the original mastectomy, that a bone scan was ordered, and they found it. I saw her suffer. By that time, my father had already passed away. He passed away in 1990, and this was 1992. We brought her home. At that time, there wasn't a Family Medical Leave Act or anything like that. She said she wanted to be with her family, so we were her caregivers. We ..." Penny's voice trailed off and she looked away.

As if she was shaking off the intrusive fear that she, too, might someday have a recurrence of one of her cancers, she said abruptly, "But I'm a fighter. I was not going to give up. I knew in my heart that God was going to take care of me. I have strength in my faith. I prayed and prayed and prayed. I had people in prayer circles praying for me. I feel truly blessed. I really do. Not only to survive the breast cancer, but the ovarian cancer on top of that. That tells me I'm blessed, and I am special. And I have a tremendous support system with family and friends."

Her support came from many sources, including women in her cancer support group, her co-workers, and a childhood friend, Cyndi, who lives in California. Most of all, though, support came from her younger sister, Kimberly Balousek, whom Penny repeatedly referred to as "my rock." Despite the many people who were eager to help her, Penny admitted that, at least initially, accepting help did not come naturally. She said, "The way I grew up, I'm a very proud person, and for my girlfriend to say, 'I'm going to take you to your chemo treatment,' was at first hard for me." Penny shook her head vigorously as she added, "I said, 'Oh, no, no. I don't need anybody to go with me.'

"My husband went with me for the first one, but my sister and my friend, Irene, actually took turns going with me from there on out. I know that he had a very hard time watching them poke me and having to watch me feel sick."

As she formed new friendships and strengthened existing ones, she began to look more closely at her relationship with her husband. They had been married for 16 years and had been to a marriage counselor even before she was diagnosed. She said, "He's not very good at showing his emotions, I would say. At the beginning, I think he was trying to ignore it—thinking maybe it would go away ... I think he thought that when I was through with chemo that everything would just go away, but it's a life-changing event. I think he thought that you could shut the door and everything would be back to the way it was." Penny paused, shook her head slowly, and bit her lip.

"I'm not back to the way I was prior to cancer. I learned to step back and evaluate things before I judge. I really learned the power of prayer and faith. I learned to depend on others a little better. I learned the true meaning of friendship.

"Steve and I got back on track for a while, but I think I totally shut down in some ways during my cancer journey. There are things that, if he were to say or do today, there would be no way I'd put up with ... Once I was finished with all my treatments and back to work, he started acting the same way and making the same comments as before. I finally sat down with him and said, 'You've got to know that I'm unhappy. You've got to see that this marriage just isn't working.'

"He went into an angry mode right away." Penny made her voice sound gruff. "'Well, okay, what do you want to do? Do you want to split up? Who gets what? Who's going to get this? Who's going to get that?' I just looked at him and said, 'I don't care.' He was missing the point totally. So I actually took our dog, Faith, and left for a while, thinking that when I came home, he'd be asleep.

"When I came home, he was still awake and said, 'Can we talk?' I said, 'Well, if you want to talk, yeah, but I'm not going to put up with the type of behavior that you showed prior to me leaving the house.' We sat down and talked—what bothered him, what bothered me. I said, 'I'm not going to live like this.'

"At first, he said, 'I'm just concerned about you. I don't want you to get sick again, and you always overexert yourself, and you take so much on your plate, doing these long hours at work again.'

"I said, 'Well, Steve, you're my partner. You're not my father, and you're treating me like your child, and I don't want a father. I *had* one ...' " Penny's voice trailed off. She cleared her throat and continued. "'I'm not going to live in the same household with a person like that. I've changed a lot, and I look at life differently. Every minute counts with me. Every minute, every second—I want to make it meaningful.' I think he got that. I think it woke him up some."

Penny grinned and raised her eyebrows. "Now, don't get me wrong. We still have days that we need to work out things, but [we agreed to] talk about it, not let it build up inside. We have a long way to go, but we are still together, and I believe that we can work on it and make it work." Penny nodded her head and smiled shyly.

"I've never understood people who complain about a problem and don't do anything about it. I had that attitude sometimes before I had cancer, but now I have the attitude that I'm fighting for my life. I'm going to make my life count. It's *my* choice whether I'm going to be miserable, or if I'm going to make the best of my life while I am still here."

———

Undoubtedly, Penny Burczyk's cancer experience lent urgency to rethinking the meaning and structure of her marriage. But then, to a greater or lesser degree, cancer jolts everyone within its reach. This, of course, is not a profound statement, but it still bears repeating in the context of the stories heard during my 3-Day adventures. Story after story had at least one element of reappraisal: of relationships, of work, of goals and priorities, of life's meaning, of relationship with God. Sometimes, the reappraisal resulted in a slow and subtle bend away from the way life was before cancer; at other times, the reappraisal resulted in a startling, action-provoking insight—what my dad always called "a burning bush," alluding to Moses' call from God to be Israel's deliverer, and the resulting change was as unexpected as a desert cloudburst.

Donna Lindsay's burning bush appeared one day in December 2003, two months after she underwent bilateral mastectomy for multifocal ductal carcinoma *in situ* (DCIS) at age 43. "After the surgery, I actually took off work and took short-term disability. It just hit me one day: I'm not going to be a regional sales director for a hospital area anymore. I'm tired of flying around the country. There's more to life than corporate America. I'm going to be a mom. I'm going to enjoy life. I'm going to help people. You know, God gave me a gift, and I'm going to help other people, and, in fact, I'm going to change my life. So I picked up the phone [to call her boss at AstraZeneca Global] and said, 'I want you to take me down a notch. Put me in a management role. Put me in the oncology area.'

"I had been Employee of the Year. I'd been in *Black Enterprise* for all the work I do. *Diversity.* I've actually been on *Oprah.* Hallmark Entertainment did two stories on my life about my adoption, but I said, 'I'm now going to enjoy life.'

"I asked the company if I could move to Houston, even though my job is out of San Antonio and Fort Worth, and they let me do it, and they paid for it, and they moved me. In February [2004], I went down to Houston and bought a house and moved. I wanted to be near Patrick [her fiancé] and my two sisters who live in Houston ... For the first time, when I went to a meeting, I was free, because I wasn't on stage. I wasn't competing for anything." Donna threw back her head and laughed. "I wasn't *competing* for *anything.* I wasn't *competing* to *do anything.*

"For years, people had been telling me, 'You work too hard. You never take time for yourself. You're just a go-go-go-getter. You're an A-plus personality. It's time to enjoy life.' I finally realized what God has been telling me but I wouldn't hear. He had to tell me in another way. So I say to people, 'You know what? God gave me a gift. It's not a bad thing.' It's a gift, because I realized I've *got* to *do something.*" Donna balled up her fists and pounded the air.

"Patrick always says to me, 'How are you so happy every day?' and I say, 'I am alive. *I am alive!* I'm thankful for everything in my life. I have a house. I have food. I have clothing. I have a job. I have a daughter. I have a wonderful family. I have friends. There is *nothing* in my life to complain about. There's nothing so horrible that I wouldn't be able to deal with it. *Nothing.*'"

I told Donna that this last statement reminded me of a stretched canvas poster that one of my younger sisters had sent me for my birthday the year before. It featured the Louisa May Alcott quote: "I am not afraid of storms for I have learned how to sail my ship." When my sister gave it to me, I was a long way from being able to declare that I wasn't afraid, so I suspected that my sister was actually trying to encourage me. I told Donna how much I admired her snappy attitude and wished that I could have been as resilient as she was.

She threw back her head and laughed again—one of her deep, bubbling laughs—and said, "Oh, honey, let me tell you about that. After the surgery [in Dallas], I went to Houston to recover at Patrick's house. My parents took my daughter to stay with them in Austin for a month—because they knew that I would want to lift her—which was devastating. Patrick practices during the day [he is a physician], and that's when it hit me. Right before I had my breasts removed, I had had a hysterectomy and oophorectomy. I was on hormones, so after the breast surgery, I had to come off the hormones, and I got so depressed. I went into a deep depression, and I didn't know what was *wrong* with me. I kept *crying*."

She shook her head and her smile faded. Her voice became somber. "So I called our EAP [employeee assistance program] line and got a counselor. I think she knew I was very upset, so they assigned me a counselor. I went to a therapist for about three months, and I was feeling much, much better. I had to talk about it because I didn't really think I had had cancer. They just took my boobs off; I didn't have cancer." Donna widened her eyes, wagged her head back and forth in an exaggerated arc, and mocked a frown. "*No-o-o-o-o.* I didn't have cancer. In fact, today, I wonder if I really had cancer. I don't know if that makes any sense. I don't know why I still think, Maybe I didn't have cancer. It's strange. Anyway, I went to counseling, and I felt much better.

"The funny thing was, I would try to talk to my sister about it—she's a managing partner in a Houston law firm—and she would say, 'What is wrong? You've already had your surgery. It's already done. You've been so strong through all of this. What's the deal?' and I would say, 'I know, but it's bothering me. I need to talk about it.'

"I didn't talk to that sister about it because she didn't really understand it. She would say, 'What's the problem? You're breaking down.' And Patrick, who's a wonderful, *awesome* man—I don't think he understood the emotional impact that [cancer] had on my life. I really don't think he does to this day. He encouraged me. He said, 'You don't have to have reconstruction,' but I said, 'For me, I have to. I have to do it for me.'

"For a month [after surgery], I never took my shirt off. I'd bathe in my shirt because I didn't want to look at myself. I just couldn't do it. I had expanders, but they had only put in 80 cc when I was in the hospital, and I had to wait three or four weeks before they could start to fill them. I was flatter than a board. One day, Patrick said, 'Take it off. We're going to stand here together and look in the mirror.' That really helped me cut through it. After that, I decided I was going to go to Victoria's Secret and get a padded bra to look normal. That lasted a day because my incisions were too fresh. So then I just said, 'Forget it. I'll be flat. It's okay.'"

Donna also talked about wrestling with the fear of recurrence. "I didn't have to have chemotherapy. I had a sentinel node biopsy—two nodes removed—and they were negative. I told my doctor, 'Please, put me on Arimidex®,' but they won't do it. They considered the hysterectomy five years' worth of hormone treatment. They said my chances of having a recurrence were very slim. I still disagree that I'm not on Arimidex®. I think at my next checkup—I go in January—I'm just going to say, 'Put me on it. What's the harm? I'd rather just take it.'"

Arimidex® (anastrozole) is one of the aromatase inhibitors, which, like tamoxifen, is a drug used for adjuvant hormonal therapy. These two classes of drug have the same goal—kill the cancer cell—but they go about it in different ways. Tamoxifen works by tricking the estrogen and progesterone receptors on breast cancer cells so that they bind to tamoxifen instead of estrogen or progesterone. This trickery interferes with the cell's growth and may cause its death. (Score one for the good guys.) On the other hand, aromatase inhibitors work by blocking the action of an enzyme—aromatase—that allows conversion of nonestrogen-like hormones to estrogen-like substances. When an aromatase inhibitor blocks this enzymatic reaction, the result is a depletion in estrogen in postmenopausal women. Hormone-sensitive breast cancers wither up and die. (Score another one for the good guys.)

Randomized clinical trials compared the outcome of postmenopausal women treated with one of three adjuvant hormone regimens: anastrozole alone, anastrozole in combination with tamoxifen, and tamoxifen alone. Preliminary results were published in 2002, and final results were published in 2005. "After a median follow-up of 68 months, anastrozole significantly prolonged disease-free survival … and significantly reduced distant metastases … and contralateral breast cancers…" The authors concluded: "Anastrozole should be the preferred initial treatment for postmenopausal women with localised hormone-receptor-positive breast cancer." (The authors are from the United Kingdom. That's why localized is spelled with an 's.')

Other aromatase inhibitors include exemestane (Aromasin®, made by Pharmacia) and toremifene citrate (Fareston®, made by Shire); however, Donna's insistence on Arimidex® may have to do with the fact that it is made by the pharmaceutical company that she works for—AstraZeneca.

"Do you know Dr. Ravdin?" she asked me.

"I know *of* him, sure. He's at our school." (I was referring to the University of Texas Health Science Center at San Antonio.)

She continued. "Yeah, well, Patrick programmed all my stuff into his model, and he said, 'Honey, you have less than a whatever percent chance of ever getting it again. Don't even worry. You've had a bilateral. You've had a hysterectomy. You're *okay*.'"

The model to which Donna was referring was the computer program, Adjuvant! Online (www.adjuvantonline.com), which was developed by Dr. Peter Ravdin and his associates to "help health professionals and patients with early cancer discuss the risks and benefits of getting additional therapy (adjuvant therapy: usually chemotherapy, hormone therapy, or both) after surgery." The program is useful for estimating "the risk of negative outcome (cancer related mortality or relapse) without systemic adjuvant therapy, ... the reduction of these risks afforded by therapy, and risks of side effects of the therapy." In short, the Ravdin software is a source to help doctors and patients get a general idea about how things are going to turn out. Donna's fiancé, an internist, used the program as a ploy to, once again, reassure her.

"But still, it doesn't connect. It's just not there." Donna slapped her temple. "I'll probably worry every day of my life. The goal is that I will get better about worrying. I want to just be free of it and not worry about it every time I get a sniffle." She laughed and said, "Like, I started having back pain, and I said to Patrick, 'Honey, I'm dying. It's spread. It's in my bone. It's gone to my *bone*. What am I going to do with my daughter?' I went out and had my will done. I had *everything* done. I put everything in a safety deposit box because I was convinced I had a recurrence in my bones.

"I'm sure Patrick thought I had lost my mind when I said, 'I've got to have a PET [positron emission tomography] scan. Right this second. Where can you get me in?' He got me in right away with one of his buddies, and I had the PET scan done, and I was fine."

I asked her if she felt foolish afterwards, and she threw back her head, shook it vigorously, and laughed. "*No,* because I still wondered if they caught it. I wondered if they really *really* looked at it like they should have. I told Patrick to *take it for a second opinion!* I said, 'Honey, I don't believe these people. I really think I need to be checked.' So I'm going to have another bone scan in January. It'll make me feel better."

Donna became serious and almost whispered, "See, I had a friend who had DCIS and she *died.* I hadn't realized that she didn't do anything about it—she just became holistic about eating well and drinking lots of water—but she *died.* Intellectually, anyway, I know that with the surgery and all, I'm okay, but I still worry about every little ache and pain, thinking maybe that it's cancer somewhere else." She laughed again and added, "My nose itches or my foot is sore, and I think, Omigod, the cancer's back ... I have an MBA [Master in Business Administration degree]. I've been in the pharmaceutical industry for 22 years. You would think that I'd know better, but it doesn't connect."

I shared my parallel story about demanding—as in, hands-on-my-hips demanding—what amounted to a restaging for breast cancer. During the summer of 2003, I felt an occasional pinching sensation in the nipple of the "bad" breast—the one in which cancer had been discovered in June 2001. It was just like the pinching sensation at the exact spot where it turned out that cancer was residing. I might not have been quite as shrill in my insistence on a battery of expensive, time-consuming, and, to be honest, nonindicated tests had I not known that local recurrences after wide local excision most often develop within two to three years after the initial diagnosis. This statistic effectively hog-tied my common sense. Similar to Donna, I pitched what amounted to a temper tantrum. And, like Donna's physician-fiancé, my physician-fiancé arranged for the tests.

We laughed at our exaggerated concern about recurrence, and we chided each other for knowing better than to insist on a study as tricky as a PET scan. (As demonstrated by Karen Schweibish's experience in the San Francisco chapter, PET scans have specific indications but should not be used as a screening test.) Donna particularly enjoyed my story because she knew my fiancé, Dr. Thomas Fisher. In fact, the reason that she was walking in Arizona—how she even *knew* about the 3-Day—was because Tom had told her about it when she called his office about 10 days prior to the event. We marveled at the sequence of events that resulted in our acquaintance, beginning with Tom's casual remark about my involvement with the event, and our chance meeting at dinner on Day 1 when she walked up to the table where I was sitting with Barbara Jo and Bob Kirshbaum in the Horizon High School gymnasium in Scottsdale.

When we first met, I was not in a very cheerful mood. In fact, I was nearly distraught. For the first time during all of the 3-Day events, I had sustained an injury that threatened to sideline me. It happened near the end of Day 1's route when I stepped off a curb and landed wrong. Although I was able to limp to camp—and avoid being swept—my foot was throbbing by the time I arrived there. Bob insisted that I stay seated, with my foot propped up, while he fetched coffee and supper for me. He then went to his car and brought back some strong medicine. Despite his and Barbara Jo's soothing words and encouragement, it was all I could do to keep from crying.

As I slouched there, foot throbbing, I muttered to myself, "I have made it 560 miles. I just *can't* be injured now. It wouldn't be *fair* if I couldn't finish." The scores of posters and banners that covered the walls of the gym, lauding the efforts of the 3-Day participants, only served to aggravate me. After all, Opening Ceremonies that morning had been

particularly meaningful for me since I had been asked by Matthew Basile—
the "voice of the 3-Day"—to deliver the Survivors' Circle speech.

Matthew was a tall, lanky man, with wavy, brown, shoulder-length
hair and an unrushed manner that belied the essentiality of his duties as
stage manager for the 3-Day. Not only did he make sure that Opening
and Closing Ceremonies and nighttime activities ran smoothly—a de-
ceptively difficult job—but he had a deep, soothing voice that matched
his easygoing demeanor. I probably wasn't the only woman at the 3-Day
who sometimes had the sensation of a warm hand on her inner thigh
when she heard Matthew's voice over the speaker. Maybe if Matthew
had been there that evening to comfort me, I wouldn't have been feeling
so defeated.

While I was working on a solid case of self-pity, Donna stopped by
our table and struck up a conversation with Barbara Jo (the 3-Day leg-
end). I didn't really pay much attention to what she and Barbara Jo were
talking about until I overheard "San Antonio." It was then that I realized
that she might be the AstraZeneca Group representative whom Tom
had mentioned. When I learned that, indeed, she was, I introduced myself. She squealed and hugged me, like we were long-lost friends. I felt
better immediately and said, "If I can walk in the morning, can I interview you for a book I'm writing?"

She flashed me one of her brilliant smiles and said, "I would *love*
to!"

As she turned to go, I remember thinking that it wasn't fair for
someone to appear so fresh and rested and to be so enthusiastic after
just walking 20 miles. I think the foot injury was making me crabby
because the next morning, with my foot well medicated (thanks to Dr.
Bob), I was not only able to keep up with Donna, but I laughed more
than I had during any of the other 3-Day interviews. My foot may not
have been hurting at the end of Day 2, but my abdomen was—from
laughing so much. And maybe I didn't notice my foot hurting because I
was so interested in her story.

Donna was born in Washington, D.C., but, because of her mother
and stepfather's doctoral studies and their subsequent teaching and educational administrative positions, she and her family (of five daughters)
moved first to Gainesville, Florida, and then to Lincoln, Nebraska. Their
final relocation was to the Northwest Hills subdivision in Austin (about 2
miles from where my family with four daughters lived in Allandale). She
attended Anderson High School (the same high school that one of my
younger sisters attended) where she was a cheerleader, and participated
in track and field, even setting a record in the long jump that held until
2004. She attended the University of Hawaii on a cheerleading scholarship but, after a year and a half, became homesick and returned to Austin where she received a bachelor's degree in clinical nutrition and bio-
chemistry from the University of Texas (where I received my bachelor's

degree in biology). Consequently, we had several miles' worth of do-you-knows and do-you-remembers.

After graduating, she moved to the Dallas area for graduate school at Texas Women's University in Denton. While she was going to school and working part time as a nutritionist at Parkland Hospital, she met her first husband, who was a surgery resident. "We dated for a few years and then decided to get married … I liked him, but I don't know if I really loved him. He just fit the mold of what my parents thought was the person I should marry: someone professional; educated; preferably a doctor, lawyer, whatever … So we got married, and we started fighting on that very day at the hotel … We just had different ways of looking at life.

"We could never come together. He lived in Boston during his residency and I lived in Washington, D.C. By then, I was working in the pharmaceutical industry, and I was supporting us because, as a resident, he didn't have a big salary. I would go visit him, maybe every six weeks … When he finished his residency and fellowship, we moved to Tulsa and he got a job with a pretty large group … When I was ready, I finally said, 'We've got to get a divorce. This is just not working.' So we divorced—which was probably the best thing—and I went on with my life. I've been divorced for 14 years.

"Then I moved to Chicago and I dated a nice guy who was never really interested in marriage and settling down. But we kept dating because it was …" Donna shrugged, and continued, "well, it was something to do. Six months after I adopted my daughter, I transferred to Texas, and he'd come and visit every now and then. I kind of got disinterested, because I had my daughter and I didn't want him to be around her. So I said to my sister, Cheryl, 'I have *got* to meet a nice man,' and she said, 'Well, you know Dr. Wills has been after you for years. I'll page him.'

"That night, he was there, all spiffed up." Donna laughed, her eyes sparkling more than usual, obviously enjoying the memory. "We sat on my sister's couch, in her living room, talking like third-graders." Pointing to the right and left, she said, "I'm right over here, and he's way over there, and we're talking—his shoes all polished—and I'm thinking, This is so corny, but I'm also thinking, Omigod, this is an *awesome, awesome* man. And I'm thinking, Ask me out for drinks! Ask me out for drinks!, but he didn't. So we shook hands and he left.

"My family's all back there, listening to us. As soon as he leaves, they all rush out asking, 'How was it? How was it?'" She rolled her eyes and said, "So he didn't call me the next day, and I'm freaking out, but he's calling my sister saying, 'What should I do? I don't want to seem too anxious. I don't want to call her too soon.' So my sister said, 'Donna, pick up the phone and call him.' But I said, 'I can't do this. Mother would *die* if she knew I did something like that. That's too *forward*.'

"I finally got up the nerve to call him, and he said, 'I was just about to call you.' We ended up having these long conversations. I'm living in Dallas, and he's in Houston, so we had all these long conversations by cell phone. He's just an awesome guy ... He has three grown daughters and, from the beginning, I let him know that I had adopted a little girl and that he had to either accept her or not and that we had to deal with it now. He loves my daughter ..." Donna's face softened and she said, softly, "Chloe. Chloe Jasmine.

"When I was younger, I never wanted kids. My first husband and I agreed that we weren't going to have kids. We were going to work. He was going to be a doctor, and I was going be a company vice president, running a company. But when I hit 30, I thought, I really want kids. At that point, I wasn't dating anyone. At 38, I thought, I *really* want to have a child, but I did nothing about it. At 41, I went into the doctor and said, 'I'm going to have *in vitro* fertilization,' but he said that my eggs were gone and that the chance of me ever getting pregnant on my own were next to nil. At that point, my younger sister stepped forward—at that time she was 32—and she took all the medication, injections, everything. She did it, and she gave me her eggs. I went through *in vitro* fertilization, and I got pregnant, but I miscarried."

In January 2002, Donna was able to adopt her daughter through an Illinois agency. She said, "It is rare that you find African-American women who are single that adopt—who go through the process. You have a lot of families in which, for instance, a woman will take her cousin's child, but it's not a legitimate adoption, through the system ... So Hallmark Entertainment contacted me about filming the process. They wanted to follow the stories of three single black women who have adopted ... Oprah decided that she was going to commend it, so we appeared on *Oprah* with the babies ... After that, we had so many women coming up to us to ask how they could adopt as single black women. The three of us will never leave each others' sides. We take the kids on a trip every year, and we will do this until they say, 'We don't want to do this anymore.'" Donna laughed again.

Her face and voice softened and she continued. "Chloe is such a pretty little girl. She's a sweetheart. Tiffany [the birth mother] and I have kept in touch. I have an open adoption, which means she can come for a visit, as long as it's supervised. Tiffany has written letters and has sent her high school graduation picture, and we've visited Tiffany at least four or five times. It's important for me to have an album for Chloe with her birth mom ... Chloe's a brilliant little girl ... She goes to a Montessori school—wears a little uniform every day. She's just the brightest little girl, the happiest little girl. I've always had a live-in nanny that helps me. She's with her this weekend. My parents just smother her, too. She's a blessed little girl."

As we parted, Donna and I arranged to meet at camp that evening so that she could say hello to Tom, who was flying in so that he could walk with me on the final day of the last 3-Day walk for 2004. Bob Kirshbaum had offered to pick up Tom at the airport that afternoon and was planning to find me along the route. Because of Tom's anticipated arrival, I had intended to walk by myself during the afternoon of Day 2; however, shortly after lunch, I spotted two women wearing Wild Women Outfitters caps—like the ones worn by the garrulous Boston 3-Day team. I caught up with them and introduced myself. It turned out that the women were sisters—Cynthia Crisp, 52, and her sister Carol Holt, both from New Hampshire. This was the third year that they were walking in 3-Day events. Their first event was in 2002, about a year after their mother was diagnosed with breast cancer. They had also walked in Washington, D.C. Arizona was their third event for 2004.

We talked about the differences in weather between the 2004 Boston event (high 80s and humid) and the Arizona event (70s and dry). We lamented the rationing of flu shots, since Cynthia was the director of employee health services at a hospital. And, since the women were from the northeast and had participated in Boston 3-Day events, we talked about the thrilling comeback of the Red Sox against the Yankees in the American League pennant race, and their prospects of winning the World Series against the St. Louis Cardinals. We chatted, in other words.

But then, out of the blue, Cynthia told me a story, which included a sentence that, when I heard it, felt like one of the desert sky's single, swift raindrops. I turned on my tape recorder and asked her if she would mind repeating the story.

She said (or, rather, repeated), "Four years ago, I knew that my sister, Christine, who was over 40, had not had a mammogram. I was very concerned about that because there's a high incidence of breast cancer in our family. One of my cousins died at 26, and my mother's own mother had breast cancer and a mastectomy. I kept asking my sister if she would go with me to have a mammogram, and she said she would, but she got busy and didn't.

"When it came time for my birthday—I always have my mammogram the month of my birthday; that way I don't forget it—she asked me what I wanted for my birthday. I knew she wouldn't refuse me, so I said, 'For my birthday, I want you to go have a mammogram with me.' I told her that I'd make the appointment.

"Then I asked my other sister, Carol, who's real good about getting her mammograms, if she'd had hers yet that year, and she said, 'No,' so I said, 'Christine and I are going. Come have yours with us.' She said, 'Sure.'

"Then I called my mom and said, 'Have you had your mammogram this year?' She said, 'Well, actually, it's been a couple of years,' and I said, 'Christine and Carol and I are all going to have a mammogram on my birthday. Will you have a mammogram with me? I'll make all the arrangements,' and she said, 'Sure.'

"So we went for our mammograms and my worst nightmare came true. My mom had breast cancer. But it was an early detection, and she didn't have to have a mastectomy, just a wide local excision—like a quarter of her breast—and all her lymph nodes removed, and she had radiation. They also wanted to do chemo, but she said that she just didn't think she could stand that. She also takes tamoxifen, but now she says that not a day goes by that she doesn't wish that she would have taken chemotherapy. She knows that that was her one shot at doing everything, and she may not get that chance again. It's been four years now. She was 68 at the time, and she's great as far as the cancer goes.

"I truly believe that early detection is what's going to save lives, and right now, the best screening test that we have is the mammogram. We make it an annual party now. I make all the appointments, and we all take the day off from work. Starting two years ago—this will be the third year—I made pink johnnies [hospital gowns] with pink feather boas for everyone. We sit in the waiting room together and take turns having our mammograms, and then we have our pictures taken. The other women who are coming in to have their mammograms always ask, 'Why can't I have a johnnie like that?' They'll look at us and say, 'I want to be part of *their* group.'" Cynthia nodded slowly, as if she had just made an important point, and added, "After we're through, we all go out to lunch and celebrate our lives.

"When my mom was diagnosed, the doctor wanted to sit down with my mom and go over all the options. We asked the doctor if the females in our family could come and listen, and she said, 'Absolutely.' We had probably 12 women in our family—even the young women and teen-agers—sitting there and listening while she went over all the options. I mean, that's part of the education, right? You're not going to get people to have their mammograms and do their self-exams if they don't know how important it is. We wanted to be certain that my mother's granddaughters understood—especially with the family history—the importance of breast self-exams and mammograms.

"My daughters are 30 and 33, and they're excited about being able to join the group soon. They say, 'Mommy, are you sure you have enough material to make our johnnies?'" Cynthia laughed and continued. "It's almost like a Ya-ya Sisterhood. I brought along one of my friends who hadn't had a mammogram in 14 years, because she was so afraid of what they might find. This will be her third year. There are eight of us now that go. It's become a fun day. Every woman talks about how they hate to have their mammograms done, but we really look forward to it. It's a social time.

"It would be great if women would take care of the other women in their lives and be certain that everybody has had their mammograms.

Oftentimes, people get caught up. They're busy and they forget. They put it off. They don't even realize how long it's been. My mom said it had been two years; it had been four years. Look at it this way: It's a gift that you're giving yourself because you're going to have that person. I still have my mom. Who knows, if she'd waited."

Before she told her story, no one had ever stated—as clearly, any-way—the most important reason to gather stories for a book. When Cynthia said, "It would be great if women would take care of the other women in their lives and be certain that everybody has had their mammograms," I knew she had said something important.

The telling of stories is, at its core, the attempt to take care of the other people in our lives. Through our stories, we share lessons and imply, "We're in this together."

About 10 months after I finished the walks, when I was nearing completion of the first draft of this story collection, my son, Andrew, phoned me, excited about a passage that he had just read in a book by Tim O'Brien entitled, *If I Die in a Combat Zone Box Me Up and Ship Me Home*. The book is a memoir about the author's year as a foot soldier in Vietnam. The quote is the last paragraph of Chapter 3:

Do dreams offer lessons? Do nightmares have themes, do we awaken and analyze them and live our lives and advise others as a result? Can the foot soldier teach anything important about war, merely for having been there. I think not. He can tell war stories.

Taken at face value, Tim O'Brien's statement is wrong, of course, because the foot soldier's war story can teach us a great deal. In fact, the more often foot soldiers tell their stories, the more likely that we can learn *everything* important about war. I realized that the situation was not unlike hearing the 3-Day stories. Although the incredible people whom I walked beside may not have aspired to teach anything important about battling cancer, they accomplished just that. They told their stories.

I had my title.

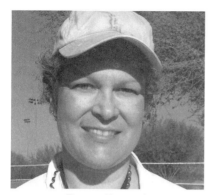

Penny Burczyk

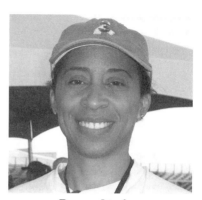

Donna Lindsay

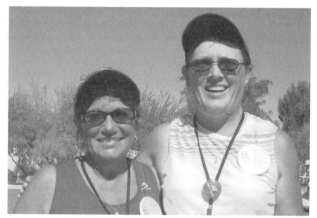

Sisters Cynthia Crisp and Carol Holt

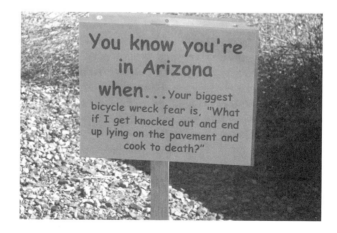

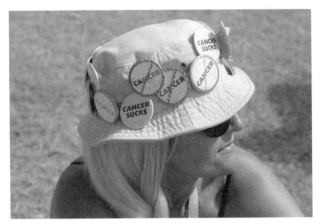

Robin Steiner

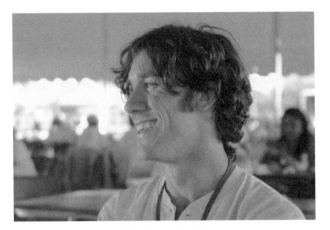

Matthew Basile

End Notes

Chapter 1

1. Pam Belluck, "To Trace Kerry's Footsteps, Get a Good Pair of Sneakers," *The New York Times*, July 25, 2004.

2. Tom Hayden, "Advice From a Veteran of the Barricades," *The New York Times*, July 25, 2004.

3. Joe Burgess, "All Roads Lead to Boston" (map), *The New York Times*, July 25, 2004.

4. Sarah Schweitzer, "For Texas Delegates, A Lonely Role," *The Boston Globe*, July 28, 2004.

5. Jennifer Stewart, "Cup and Saucer" (www.cupandsaucer.com/blog), "Just the FAQ's Ma'am!" Her current Web site is www.jenstewart.com.

6. Frances Hodgson Burnett, *The Secret Garden* (London: William Heinemann, 1911).

7. Jennifer Stewart, "Cup and Saucer" (www.cupandsaucer.com/blog), "Cranky, Cranky, Cranky," September 19, 2003.

8. Ibid., "For the Sake of Context ...," July 5, 2003.

9. Ibid., "Whatcha See Is, Well, Whatcha Get," October 29, 2003.

10. Ibid., "Getting Healthy ... One Day at a Time" (opening page to "Jen's Breast Cancer Page").

11. Team Wild Women Originals (www.teamwork.com).

12. Men With Heart (www.menwithheart.org).

Chapter 2

1. Cabaret Theatre of Rutgers University (www.cabaret-theatre.org), "Cabaret Theatre's 'Where Are They Now?'"

2. Christina Jeng, "Reopened Lady Liberty Welcomes Back Hundreds," *USA Today*, August 4, 2004.

Chapter 3

1. National Aeronautics and Space Administration (www.nasa.gov/vision/ universe/watchtheskies/25jun), "The 2004 Perseid Meteor Shower."

2. L.P. Middleton, M. Amin, K. Gwyn, et al., "Breast carcinoma in pregnant women: assessment of clinicopathologic and immunohistochemical features," *Cancer* 98:1055-1060, 2003.

3. L.A. Emens and N.E. Davidson, "The follow-up of breast cancer," *Seminars in Oncology* 30:338-348, 2003.

4. Carolynn Johnson, "Pink Ribbon Miracle" (www.pinkribbonmiracle.com), "Friday, June 4, 2004."

5. Ibid., "Tuesday, June 22, 2004."

6. Young Survival Coalition® (www.youngsurvival.org).

Chapter 4

1. K.A. Skinner, J.T. Helsper, D. Deapen, et al., "Breast cancer: do specialists make a difference?" *Annals of Surgical Oncology* 10:606-615, 2003.

2. Elizabeth Naftalis, "Breast cancer: do specialists make a difference?" *Breast Diseases: A Year Book® Quarterly* 15:18, 2004.

3. K.A. Phillips, R.L. Milne, M.L. Friedlander, et al., "Prognosis of premenopausal breast cancer and childbirth prior to diagnosis," *Journal of Clinical Oncology* 22:699-705, 2004.

4. G.H. Lyman, D.C. Dale, and J. Crawford, "Incidence and predictors of low dose-intensity in adjuvant breast cancer chemotherapy: a nationwide study of community practices," *Journal of Clinical Oncology* 21:4524-4531, 2003.

5. Nick Bunkley, "Woodward Dream Cruise," *The Detroit News*, August 18, 2004.

6. P.K. Rauch, A.C. Muriel, and N.H. Cassem, "Parents with cancer: who's looking after the children?" *Journal of Clinical Oncology* 20(21):4399-4402, 2002.

7. Henry Ford Health System (www.henryford.com).

Chapter 5

1. Grant Wahl, "Out of this World," CNN/Sports Illustrated (http://sportsillustrated.cnn.com/soccer/world/1999/womens), issued July 19, 1999, posted July 23, 1999.

2. Betty Friedan, *The Feminine Mystique* (New York: W.W. Norton & Company, 1963).

3. M.L. Citron, D.A. Berry, C. Cirrincione, et al., "Randomized trial of dose-dense versus conventionally scheduled and sequential versus concurrent combination chemotherapy as postoperative adjuvant treatment of node-positive primary breast cancer: first report of Intergroup Trial C9741/Cancer and Leukemia Group B Trial 9741," *Journal of Clinical Oncology* 21:1431-1439, 2003.

Chapter 6

1. C.K. Raymond, S. Subramanian, M. Paddock, et al., "Targeted, haplotype-resolved resequencing of long segments of the human genome," *Genomics* 86(6):759-766, 2005.

2. Jimmie C. Holland and Sheldon Lewis, *The Human Side of Cancer: Living with Hope, Coping with Uncertainty* (New York: HarperCollins, 2000), pp. 14-15.

3. John Doman, "Showing Off" (photograph caption), *St. Paul Pioneer Press*, September 13, 2004.

Chapter 7

1. I.J. Lerner and B.J. Kennedy, "The prevalence of questionable methods of cancer treatment in the United States," *CA: A Cancer Journal for Clinicians* 42:181-191, 1992.

2. Richard and Annette Bloch, *Cancer ... There's Hope* (The R.A. Bloch Cancer Foundation, Inc., 1982).

3. A. Liede, B.Y. Karlan, R.L. Baldwin, et al., "Cancer incidence in a population of Jewish women at risk of ovarian cancer," *Journal of Clinical Oncology* 20:1570-1577, 2002.

4. Canine Companions for Independence (www.caninecompanions.org).

Chapter 8

1. John Ritter, "St. Helens Closer to Big Eruption," *USA Today*, October 4, 2004.

2. Hester Hill Schnipper, *After Breast Cancer: A Common-Sense Guide to Life After Treatment* (New York: Bantam Books, 2003), p. 14.

3. The GIVIO Investigators, "Impact of follow-up testing on survival and health-related quality of life in breast cancer patients: a multicenter randomized controlled trial," *Journal of the American Medical Association* 271(20):1587-1592, 2004.

4. M.R. del Turco, D. Palli, A. Cariddi, et al., "Intensive diagnostic follow-up after treatment of primary breast cancer: a randomized trial," *Journal of the American Medical Association* 271(20):1593-1597, 1994.

5. Lance Armstrong and Sally Jenkins, *It's Not About the Bike: My Journey Back to Life* (New York: Putnam, 2000).

6. Pink Wings 4 Breast Cancer (www.pinkwings.com).

7. The Susan G. Komen Breast Cancer Foundation (www.komen.org).

Chapter 9

1. Healing Odyssey (www.healingodyssey.org).

2. Warming Hut Hotties (www.warminghuthotties.com).

Chapter 10

1. Sara Thorson, "'Winter' weather on the way to Arizona," *East Valley Tribune*, October 21, 2004.

2. Eva S. Singletary, editor-in-chief, *Breast Diseases: A Year Book® Quarterly* (Philadelphia: Mosby, Inc.).

3. G.S. Dite, M.A. Jenkins, M.C. Southey, et al., "Familial risks, early-onset breast cancer, and *BRCA1* and *BRCA2* mutations," *Journal of the National Cancer Institute* 95:448-457, 2003.

4. M. Mahue-Giangreco, G. Ursin, J. Sullivan-Halley, et al., "Induced abortion, miscarriage, and breast cancer risk in young women," *Cancer Epidemiology Biomarkers & Prevention* 12:209-214, 2003.

5. L.M. Newcomer, P.A. Newcomb, A. Trentham-Dietz, et al., "Oral contraceptive use and risk of breast cancer by histologic type," *International Journal of Cancer* 106:961-964, 2003.

6. N. Siegelmann-Danieli, A. Tamir, H. Zohar, et al., "Breast cancer in women with recent exposure to fertility medications is associated with poor prognostic features," *Annals of Surgical Oncology*, 10:1031-1038, 2003.

7. A.S. Malin, D. Qi, X-O. Shu, et al., "Intake of fruits, vegetables and selected micronutrients in relation to the risk of breast cancer," *International Journal of Cancer* 105:413-418, 2003.

8. P. Reynolds, S. Hurley, D.E. Goldberg, et al., "Active smoking, household passive smoking, and breast cancer: evidence from the California teachers study," *Journal of the National Cancer Institute* 96:29-37, 2004.

9. C. Stahlburg, A.T. Pederson, E. Lynge, et al., "Increased risk of breast cancer following different regimens of hormone replacement therapy frequently used in Europe," *International Journal of Cancer* 109:721-727, 2004.

10. K.B. Michels and A. Ekbom, "Caloric restriction and incidence of breast cancer," *The Journal of the American Medical Association* 291:1226-1230, 2004.

11. H.S. Feigelson, C.R. Jonas, L.R. Teras, et al., "Weight gain, body mass index, hormone replacement therapy, and postmenopausal breast cancer in a large prospective study," *Cancer Epidemiology Biomarkers & Prevention* 13:220-224, 2004.

12. L. Keinan-Boker, Y.T. van Der Schouw, D.E. Grobbee, et al., "Dietary phytoestrogens and breast cancer risk," *American Journal of Clinical Nutrition* 79:282-288, 2004.

13. E. Cho, D. Spiegelman, D.J. Hunter, et al., "Premenopausal dietary intake, glycemic index, glycemic load, and fiber in relation to risk of breast cancer," *Cancer Epidemiology Biomarkers & Prevention* 12:1153-1158, 2003.

14. L.G. Rodriquez and A. Gonzalez-Perez, "Risk of breast cancer among users of aspirin and other anti-inflammatory drugs," *British Journal of Cancer* 91:525-529, 2004.

15. K.B. Michels, S.E. Hankinson, C.G. Solomon, et al., "Type 2 diabetes and subsequent incidence of breast cancer in the nurses' health study," *Diabetes Care* 26:1752-1758, 2003.

16. M. Baum, A.U. Budzar, J. Cuzick, et al., "Anastrozole alone or in combination with tamoxifen versus tamoxifen alone for adjuvant treatment of postmenopausal women with early breast cancer: first results of the ATAC randomized trial," *Lancet* 359(9324):2131-2139, 2002.

17. A. Howell, J. Cuzick, M. Baum, et al., "Results of the ATAC (Arimidex, tamoxifen, alone or in combination) trial after completion of 5 years' adjuvant treatment for breast cancer," *Lancet* 365(9453):60-2, 2005.

18. Peter Ravdin's Adjuvant! Online (www.adjuvantonline.com).

19. Tim O'Brien, *If I Die in a Combat Zone Box Me Up and Ship Me Home* (New York: Random House, Inc., 1975), pp. 22-23.

Index

About the Author

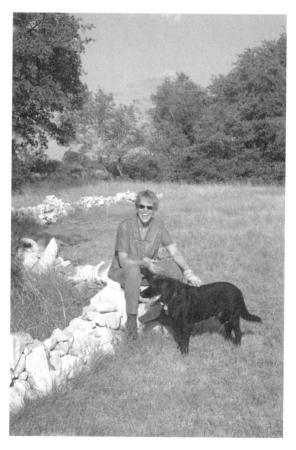

Retired pathologist, Deborah Douglas, M.D., is the author of two regional titles: the award-winning book, *Gone for the Day: Family Fun in
Central Texas*, and *Stirring Prose: Cooking with Texas Authors*, which
was cited in *DLB Yearbook 1998* in "The Year in Texas Literature" and
endorsed by First Lady Laura Bush. Dr. Douglas was diagnosed with
breast cancer in 2001 and retired a year later to devote all of her time to
writing. She recently moved to a ranch 10 miles from Burnet, Texas,
where she builds rock walls and grows organic vegetables.

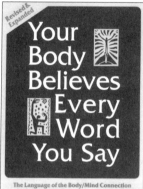
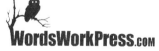